PRIMAL HEALTH DESIGN

7 KEY PARADIGMS TO REVERSE BIOLOGICAL AGE

PRIMAL

7 KEY PARADIGMS TO REVERSE BIOLOGICAL AGE

HEALTH

DR. KAVIN MISTRY

DESIGN

MUNN AVENUE PRESS

Primal Health Design

7 Key Paradigms to Reverse Biological Age

By Dr. Kavin Mistry

First Edition

Copyright © 2025 by Dr. Kavin Mistry

Published by

Munn Avenue Press

300 Main Street, Ste 21

Madison, NJ 07940

MunnAvenuePress.com

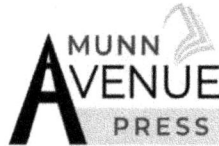

Illustrations: Tracey Porter (Pixeleiderdown)

Cover Design: Aksharamantra

ISBN Hardcover: 978-1-960299-83-3

ISBN Paperback: 978-1-960299-82-6

Printed in the United States of America

Dedication

To my beloved parents,
Dalpat and Sudha Mistry,

For your unwavering love, quiet strength, and timeless wisdom. You taught me the value of integrity, purpose, and grace—and planted the seeds of curiosity, resilience, and devotion that shaped every chapter of my life.

This book is for you.

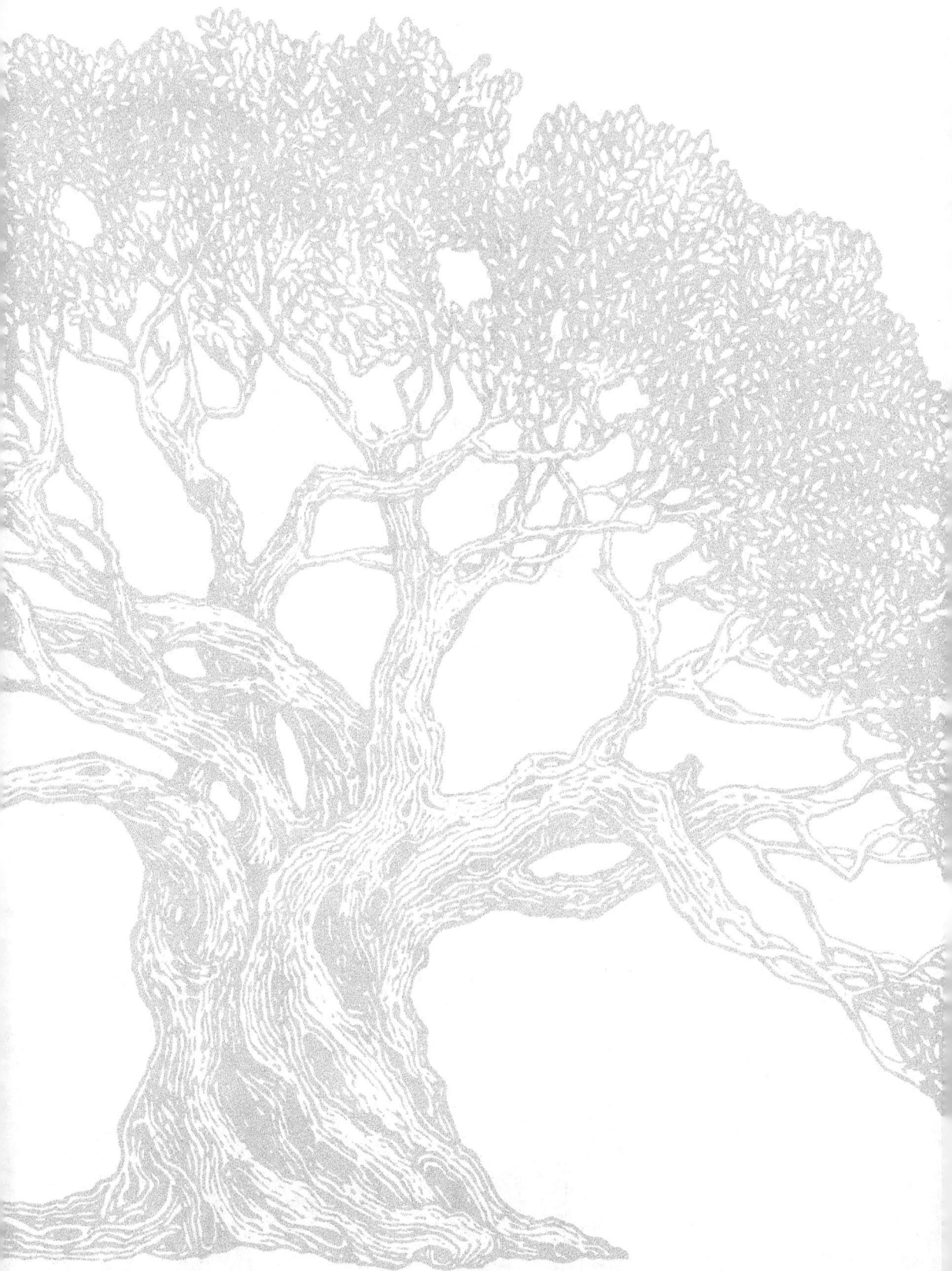

CONTENTS

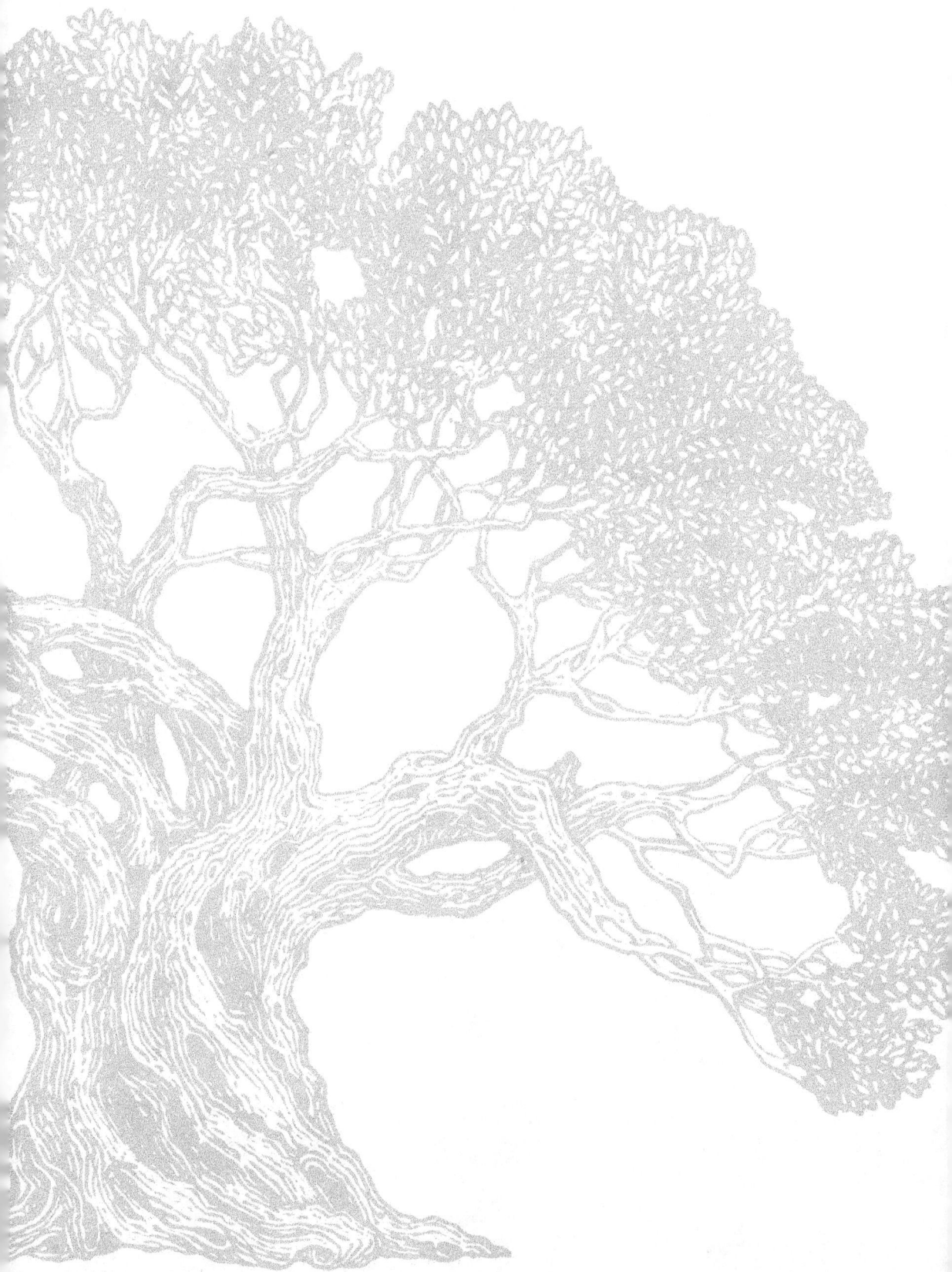

INTRODUCTION

It was the summer of 1999, and the hospital corridors hummed softly with fluorescent lights, an eerie soundtrack to the night. As a first-year resident at Robert Wood Johnson University Hospital in New Jersey, sleep was a rare luxury, and on-call shifts blurred into endless rounds of beeping monitors and distant alarms.

At 3:00 a.m., the overhead speaker shattered the silence with an urgent code alert, yanking me from the edge of sleep into harsh reality. Adrenaline surged through me, propelling me into action before my thoughts could gather. I hit the cold floor, fumbling for the code cart, my mind foggy from stolen minutes of sleep. The hallway seemed to stretch forever as I raced to the patient's room, struggling to focus.

I burst into the room amid a storm of activity. The attending cardiologist, steadfast and stern, was rhythmically compressing the patient's chest at the bedside. Harsh light cast shadows that danced on the walls, and the cardiologist's grunts punctuated the relentless beeping of the heart monitor, a haunting reminder of time slipping away.

The patient, a 37-year-old man, lay lifeless amid the chaos. The attending physician's frustration was palpable, a blend of determination and desperation. Swiftly, he took the code cart from me, deftly preparing the defibrillator. When the paddles pressed against the patient's chest, I braced for impact.

The first shock sent the patient's body into a grotesque convulsion, but the monitor's flatline persisted, blunt and unyielding. "Come on, man, come on," the cardiologist urged, as if willing the heart back to life. The second shock followed, more forceful, yet the body settled again, lifeless. The line remained stubbornly flat, echoing finality.

By the third shock, tension suffocated the room. The doctor's hands trembled slightly as he delivered the final jolt. The body jerked once more, then fell still. Silence enveloped us, broken only by the monotony of the flatline. The cardiologist, weighed down by defeat, turned to us, his voice heavy with exhaustion, and said, "Go talk to the family."

Rooted to the spot, the thought of facing the young wife and her two toddlers was unbearable. I let the others go; my legs felt like lead as I returned to my call room. The dim space, once a refuge, now felt like a prison. I sat on the edge of the bed, head in hands, replaying the events over and over.

Frustration boiled within me, frustration at the limits of modern medicine, at our inability to save a young man. Anger followed, sharp and raw. How could his health deteriorate so much? How could I feel so powerless as a doctor?

As the anger faded, more profound questions emerged: How do I move forward? How do I grow from this? That night marked the beginning of a journey to question the foundation of our healthcare system. Given the right conditions, I realized that our bodies have an innate ability to heal. Yet modern society often obstructs this process.

Over the past 25 years, I've sought answers, explored new paradigms, and gathered scientific truths. This book is the culmination of that journey, starting that summer night in 1999. I share these insights with great pride, hoping we can rediscover the essence of primal health, longevity, and abundant energy together.

There Is Still Time. Turn Around.

Two priests stood steadfast beside a winding bridge on a dark, stormy night. Their robes flapped in the wind as they held up signs that read, "There is still time. Turn around."

As the stormy night deepened, a pickup truck barreled toward them, headlights cutting through the gloom. The driver, spotting the priests, leaned out of his window and bellowed, "Leave me alone, you religious freaks!" and sped past them into the abyss.

Calmly, Father Benedict turned to his companion, a wry smile twitching at the corners of his lips. "Walter," he remarked, "maybe we need a more direct approach." He paused, listening to the echo of the engine fade into the night, replaced by an unsettling silence. "Something like, 'The bridge is out; you will die!'"

In our journey through life, we face a similar truth: The bridge is out, and the reality is that none of us are getting out of this game alive. Yet, even if we cannot change our ultimate destination, we have a choice about how we travel. Are we merely racing toward the end, or are we savoring the views along the way, genuinely experiencing the riches of life, such as health and joy? This book is not here to take you off the road but to help you slow down to enjoy the journey with vigor and presence. Our goal is to enhance your healthspan so that the road is filled with enriching and fulfilling experiences, granting you a ride worth taking.

Lifespan Versus Healthspan

As we navigate the winding road of life, it's essential to understand the distinction between lifespan and healthspan. While lifespan refers to the number of years we live, healthspan emphasizes the quality of those years, that is, how long we remain healthy, active, and able to enjoy the world around us.

In the early 1900s, the average lifespan was significantly shorter than it is today. At the turn of the century, life expectancies hovered around 47 years in the United States, primarily due to infectious diseases, a lack of modern medical care, and higher infant mortality rates. Fast-forward to the present day, and we find that advances in medicine, technology, and public health have extended our average lifespan to about 77 years. This leap forward seems astonishing at face value, a testament to human ingenuity and progress.

However, the story shifts when we scrutinize the quality of these extended years. While we live longer, we aren't necessarily living better. Rates of obesity, heart disease, cancer, high blood pressure, diabetes, and mental disorders like depression and anxiety have soared since the early 1900s. For instance, obesity, a relatively rare condition in 1900, now affects about 40.3% of adults in the U.S., according to the CDC. Heart disease and cancer, while becoming more treatable, remain the leading causes of death today, partly due to lifestyle factors that also contribute to high blood pressure and diabetes.

A particularly troubling aspect of modern life is the rising rate of mental health issues. Depression and anxiety, almost invisible in early 20th-century statistics due only in part to lack of reporting and understanding, have become prevalent, with nearly one in five adults in the U.S. experiencing mental health disorders today. Even more stark is the increase in suicide rates; the enormity of this issue is underscored by the fact that suicide, a rare tragedy in the 1900s, is now one of the leading causes of death, particularly among young people.

Interestingly, in the early 1900s, people may have had fewer chronic ailments plaguing their later years despite the shorter lifespan. The extended lifespans we enjoy now often involve years of managing chronic conditions, which detract from the quality of life in our senior years.

This is where the concept of healthspan becomes critical. To truly benefit from our increased lifespan, our focus should shift toward enhancing the healthspan, ensuring that our later years are not just long but also fulfilling, vibrant, and disease-free. It's about living with vitality, minimizing disease burden, maintaining functional abilities, and enjoying life until the end.

As we confront these challenges, this book aims to provide the tools and insights needed to extend your healthspan. By focusing on healthspan, we aim to empower you not just to add years to your life but life to your years, ensuring that you can savor every moment, experience joy, and continue to contribute to the world in meaningful ways.

Modern Man and Ancient Genes

To truly appreciate the marvel of human evolution, let's embark on a brief journey through time, tracing our lineage back through millennia to grasp the short blip of modern comforts in our existence. Homo sapiens, as a species, have roamed this earth for approximately 300,000 years. For the vast majority of this time, we thrived without the conveniences of electricity, climate control, cars, or glowing screens.

Enter the modern age: Electricity was harnessed in the late 1800s, cars arrived at the turn of the 20th century, and the first computers began blinking in the mid-20th century. In roughly a century, the entirety of our existence shifted dramatically as these advancements settled our lives in comfort.

While these technologies have improved many aspects of our lives, they have dulled the environmental stimuli that helped shape our resilience and health. Enter *epigenetics*, the study of how our environment can switch genes on and off, affecting our health and longevity over time. This field explains how external factors can influence our genes' expression without changing our DNA sequence, impacting everything from metabolism to immunity.

Imagine a day in the life of a modern human: You wake from a deep sleep in a climate-controlled cocoon atop a mattress that knows every contour of your body. Breakfast is a quick affair: packaged cereal and milk poured from a carton. You slip on your air-cushioned sneakers and step into your climate-controlled car, insulated from the weather's whims.

Your day unfolds in a plush office chair amidst the climate-controlled calm of your workspace, sheltered from the sun, the soil, and the elements that shaped our ancestors. Eight to nine hours pass in this ergonomic enclave before you return home to rinse and repeat. This cycle of comfort cocoons us from the natural world that forged our ancestral vitality.

Human bodies evolved through exposure to the raw elements as we endured fluctuations of hot and cold, moved and grounded on the earth's surface, and soaked in the sun's radiant energy. These environmental challenges shaped our biology and influenced our genes and health.

This disconnect from natural stimuli is more than just a loss of primal experience; it disrupts the signals that once ensured robust health. Lack of sunlight alters circadian rhythms, absence of temperature variation weakens our adaptive resilience, and deficiency of natural movement inhibits our functional strength.

As this book unfolds, we'll explore ways to reconnect with these ancestral environments, bringing the fundamental elements that can transform our lives back into focus. Reintegrating natural stimuli helps recalibrate our epigenetic switches, turning back the clock on modern discontent and steering us toward the vibrant health we were born to experience. The goal is not to abandon the comforts of modern life but to harmonize them with the whispers of our evolutionary past.

Crafting Health: The Journey to Designing Wellness

Life's journey often leads us back to our beginnings, asking us to rethink, reshape, and recreate our understanding of the world. My path has been no different; it has been a seamless blend of ancient traditions and modern sciences converging into a singular philosophy: **Primal Health Design.**

I come from a proud lineage of master woodworkers, a heritage embedded in my name, Mistry, meaning woodworker. For generations, my family has honored the spirit of each tree, crafting furniture that celebrated its natural form and function. In our tradition, trees were never hastily cut down. Instead, we gathered old trees, revealing the rich stories within their rings, each a lifetime recorded in the grain. Each piece of wood held an inner beauty waiting to be revealed, much like the beauty within us.

When I was five, my father's work brought us to Africa. My childhood in Africa was a vivid canvas painted with experiences that shaped my understanding of humanity and connection. My father, a civil engineer working on a World Bank project under the UN, was stationed in Arusha, Tanzania, mere miles from the breathtaking Serengeti Plateau. This proximity allowed me to engage with diverse tribal cultures, particularly the Hadzabe, or Wahadzabe, in Swahili. The Hadzabe people have inhabited the region surrounding Lake Eyasi for thousands of years, a remarkable stretch of time that intertwines their heritage with the very fabric of the Great Rift Valley, which is Africa's most biologically diverse region.

The Hadzabe are among the few remaining hunter-gatherer populations on Earth, with minimal alterations to their way of life until the last century. Living in camps of 20 to 30, their social structures are egalitarian, reflecting a sense of community that contrasts with the hierarchies often found in modern society. Their diet, rich in honey, tubers, fruits, and meat, showcases their intimate relationship with the land. The Hadza language, known as Hadzane, features unique click sounds and is unrelated to any other known language, much like their distinct way of life. As of 2015, only about 1,200 to 1,300 Hadza people remain, testifying to their resilience despite the challenges they face in a rapidly changing world.

I saw an illuminating contrast among tribes like the Hadzabe. They had minimal chronic illnesses or degenerative diseases like ours, and they lived deeply connected to the earth and each other. Those interactions etched a profound lesson into my being: Health isn't about band-aid solutions but about returning to simpler connections, connections with land, purpose, and community.

This understanding of health, fused with my family's woodworking heritage, sparked a question: **What if we could design daily practices to foster connections between earth, body, mind, and purpose, thereby counteracting the effects of modern life and transforming our health?** Could we craft a roadmap to health that guides individuals who feel lost in today's fast-paced world back to their authentic selves?

Radiologist's Perspective: Chronological vs. Biological Age

As a neuroradiologist, I have the unique privilege and responsibility of peering beneath the skin to view the ticking clock of a person's biological age. Sometimes, this age is starkly different from their chronological age. I often tell people, "You can lie about your age, but your body doesn't lie to me on my screen."

Imaging studies reveal many indicators of health and vitality. When I'm on call and evaluating an emergency room trauma study, the imaging stack typically includes CT scans of the head, cervical spine, chest, abdomen, and pelvis. Occasionally, stroke trauma cases contain even more data, including CT angiograms of the head and neck. This extensive imaging reveals much about the person's biological age.

For instance, cardiovascular health is visible in the degree of atherosclerosis: a simple glance at the aorta or cardiac vessels reveals years of dietary and lifestyle choices. Bone density and the degree of degenerative changes reveal skeletal health. The brain's volume and any evidence of past strokes or cranial trauma give insight into the individual's cognitive health. The lung windows show the person's pulmonary capacity and vitality.

My subspecialty in neuroradiology allows me to explore neurodegenerative diseases more deeply. I use tools such as functional MRI (fMRI), Diffusion Tensor Imaging (DTI), Volumetric MRI, Brain SPECT (Single Photon Emission Computed Tomography), and amyloid-targeted imaging to gain insight into issues of memory and cognition.

I recently had a case of a 48-year-old woman with a strong family history of Alzheimer's disease who presented with progressive memory loss. She started forgetting where she parked, put her keys, etc. Conventional MRI scans revealed no significant findings. However, using advanced volumetric imaging with AI processing, such as NeuroQuant, we could detect a significant decline in her hippocampal volume (an area of the brain critical in memory function) compared to previous studies, indicating a different situation. While there is an expected age-related rate of decline in some areas of the brain, like the hippocampus, this patient's decline was significantly advanced. These modern imaging tools are paving the way for earlier detection of neurodegenerative diseases and opening opportunities for earlier intervention.

This ability to gain insight into physiological age with imaging tools strengthens the emerging comprehensive biological aging model, which incorporates multiple domains, including:

1. Cellular Health: Mitochondrial function is critical for cell energy production, while the accumulation of senescent cells (those that no longer divide) accelerates aging and impacts overall health.

2. Systemic Inflammation: Chronic inflammation can disrupt cellular processes and is linked to various diseases. It acts like a silent saboteur in the body.

3. Metabolic Health: Insulin sensitivity is a key marker of metabolic flexibility. It enables the body to utilize glucose and fats for energy efficiently, maintaining balance in metabolic processes.

4. Oxidative Stress: Occurs when the body's free radicals and antioxidants are imbalanced. This leads to cellular damage and contributes to aging and disease progression.

5. Hormone Levels: Proper hormonal balance regulates many bodily functions, including metabolism, growth, and mood, making it essential for overall health as we age.

6. Gut Microbiome Diversity: A diverse gut microbiome is crucial for digestion, immunity, and even mental health, as these trillions of bacteria work in concert to influence our well-being.

7. Functional Age: Metrics such as VO2 max, muscle mass, strength, and bone density provide a comprehensive view of an individual's physical capabilities and health status, often referred to as functional age.

8. Epigenetic Flexibility: This refers to how well genes can adapt to lifestyle and environmental changes, allowing modifications to enhance resilience and health.

9. Cognitive Reserve: Cognitive reserve reflects the brain's resilience achieved through lifelong learning, social engagement, and intellectual activity, contributing to coping with damage or decline.

10. Immunosenescence: This gradual decline in immune function is influenced by aging and lifestyle choices and increases vulnerability to infections and diseases as one ages.

In piecing together this biological mosaic, we advance our understanding of aging, transforming it from mere chronology to a tailored health narrative. With these insights, we can better guide individuals in nurturing their health holistically, providing a roadmap for extending both lifespan and healthspan.

The Race That Defines Legends

Since 1923, the 24 Hours of Le Mans has been motorsports' ultimate test of endurance, speed, and strategy. Held annually in France, this legendary race pushes machines and humans to their absolute limits. Unlike conventional racing, where raw speed alone determines the victor, Le Mans demands more—engineering precision, mental resilience, and relentless teamwork. Winning isn't just about crossing the finish line first; it's about keeping the car alive for 24 punishing hours, navigating the balance between risk and preservation, and synchronizing a crew to perform with clockwork efficiency.

The team that triumphs at Le Mans excels in four key areas:

1. Mechanical Mastery – The car must survive the grueling distance. The engine, brakes, shocks, and aerodynamics must be meticulously maintained to ensure efficiency and longevity.

2. Mental Resilience – Drivers must know when to push the car to its limits and when to conserve energy. The race is a marathon, not a sprint.

3. Teamwork & Strategy – Three drivers rotate behind the wheel, relying on a pit crew that executes rapid-fire repairs and refueling. Precision and trust are paramount.

4. The Will to Win – Beyond strategy and mechanics, the defining factor is an unbreakable will to finish strong. Without it, even the best-engineered machine and the smartest team will fail.

The Le Mans of Life

Now, shift your perspective from the Circuit de la Sarthe to the grand race we're all running: **life itself.**

From childhood, we're given a script: study hard, land a good job, and you'll be set for success. But by the time most people hit their late 30s or early 40s, they realize a sobering truth: this was just the first half of the race. At 40, you're not at the finish line; you're at halftime. And like Le Mans, life is a race of endurance, not a quick sprint to an early peak.

Winning the **Le Mans of Life** requires the same four principles that determine victory on the track:

1. Physical Health: The Engine That Must Last

Your body is your race car, lasting *80 to 100 years.* Muscle mass, cardiovascular endurance (VO2 max), and joint integrity are your tires, fuel efficiency, and suspension. Without them, you won't survive the entire distance.

2. Mental Health: The Driver's Mindset

Mental acuity and resilience determine how well one navigates stress, setbacks, and life's high-speed corners. The ability to remain still in chaos, adapt, and focus separates the elite from the exhausted.

3. Emotional Health: The Pit Crew of Connection

No driver wins alone. Meaningful relationships—your partner, tribe, and purpose—are your pit crew. Without deep connections, life becomes a lonely, mechanical grind, and burnout is inevitable.

4. Existential Health: The Legacy Lap

The greatest drivers don't race just to win, they race to be remembered. A legacy mindset means working on things that outlive you, whether raising children, building something meaningful, or influencing the world beyond your years. It's the final piece that turns a life well-lived into a life well-spent.

Primal Design

In a world that often compartmentalizes health into neat little boxes, nutrition here, exercise there, and mental well-being somewhere else, **Primal Design** invites us to embrace winning the race of life. Drawing inspiration from my interactions with primal cultures in Africa, my Eastern heritage, and the nuances of modern medicine, I've come to understand that optimal health is not a single-dimensional pursuit. Instead, it combines physical, mental, emotional, and existential components harmoniously.

Physical Health: Grounding in the Earth, Food, and Our Bodies

Mental Health: The Mind-Body Connection

Emotional Health: Discovering Your Purpose and Tribe

Existential Health: Embracing Our Finiteness in an Infinite Cosmos

By nurturing these pillars, we create a robust framework for holistic well-being that honors our totality as human beings. Let's remember the interconnectedness of these facets, embracing the wisdom of primal practices while honoring the gifts of modern understanding. When we cultivate a rich experience of life—grounded in the Earth, aware of our thoughts, fueled by purpose, and accepting of our finite nature—we open the door to a more vibrant, fulfilled existence.

Primal Design

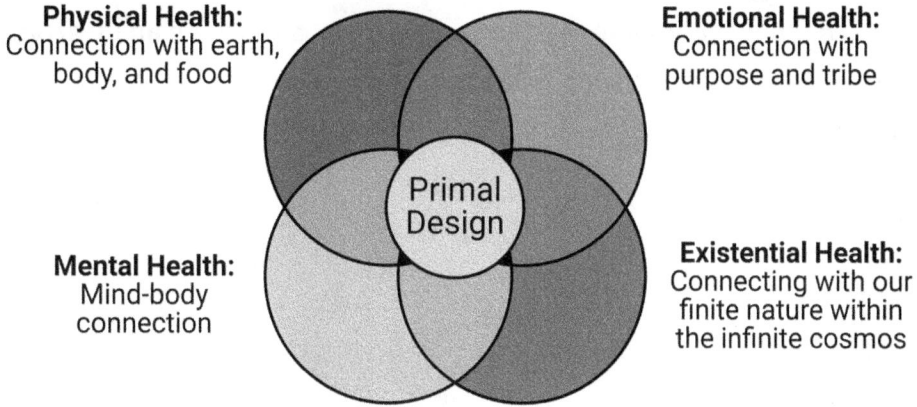

Physical Health:
Connection with earth, body, and food

Emotional Health:
Connection with purpose and tribe

Primal Design

Mental Health:
Mind-body connection

Existential Health:
Connecting with our finite nature within the infinite cosmos

Your Guide to Victory

In our pursuit of a rich and fulfilling life, we find that mere life extension isn't the ultimate goal; the quality, depth, and vibrancy of each moment truly matter. *Primal Health Design* offers a race strategy for the Le Mans of Life, guiding you to maintain your physical machine, sharpen your mental reflexes, fuel your emotional connections, and build a legacy worth leaving behind. Because when the checkered flag falls, true success is not merely measured by the distance traveled but by the grace and wisdom with which you journeyed.

Primal Health Design is more than a blueprint for reversing biological aging or fostering holistic wellness; it is a call to reconnect with the essence that sustains us. With its foundational paradigms, specifically, connecting with the earth, embracing vitalizing foods, honing physical and mental acuity, discovering purpose and community, and reconciling our finite existence within an infinite cosmos, we embark on a journey to extend life and fill it with connection and clarity. We awaken our primal vitality and rediscover the dormant wisdom, rekindling our innate health intelligence.

In an era when modern society has distanced us from the sources of life, vibrancy, and resilience, *Primal Health Design* emerges as a collective movement, a unifying force for reclaiming our health and rediscovering our ancient wisdom. **This path to wellness is not an external quest; it's an internal one, guiding us to reconnect with what is primal, what is real, and what truly sustains us.**

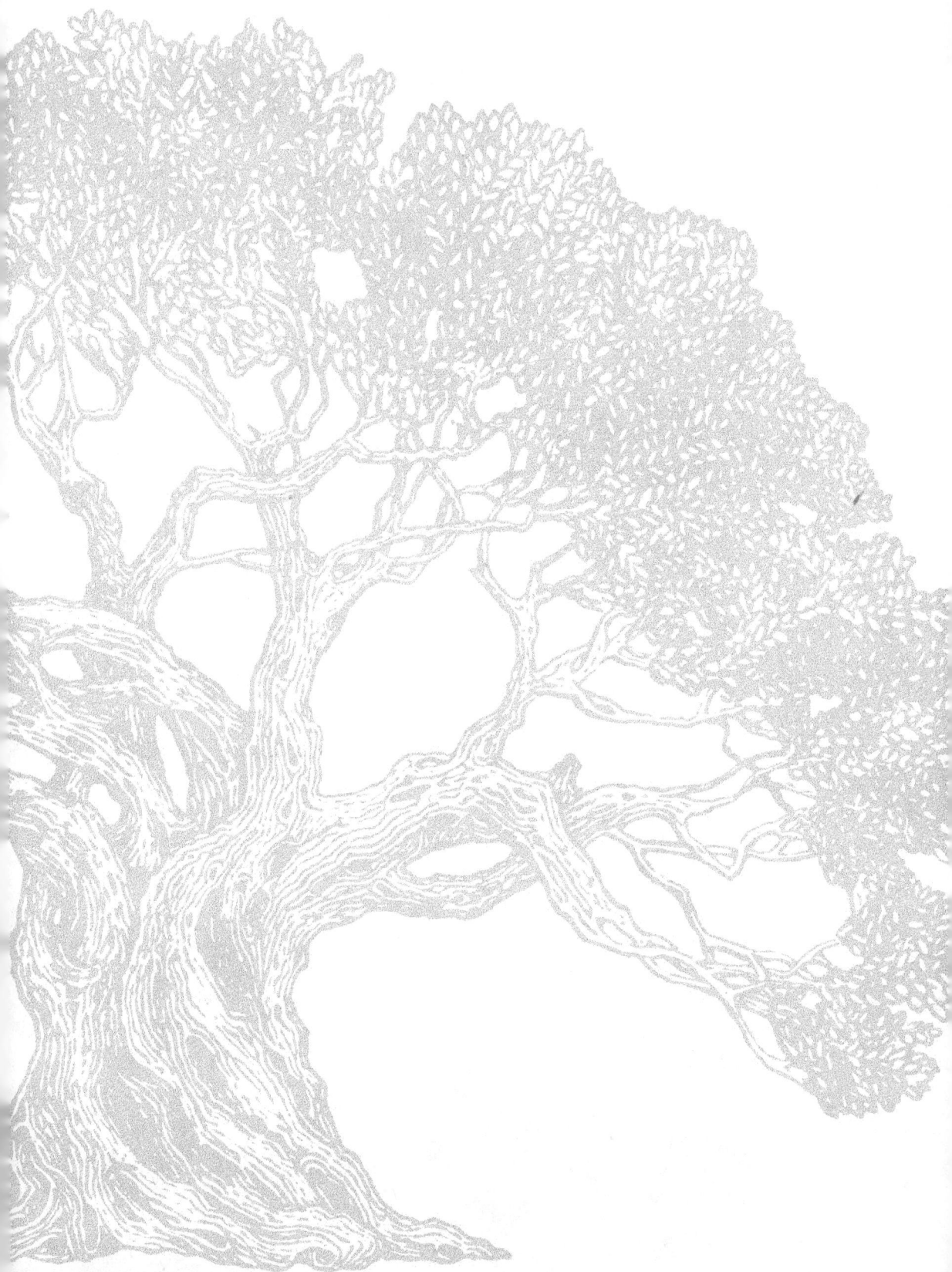

1

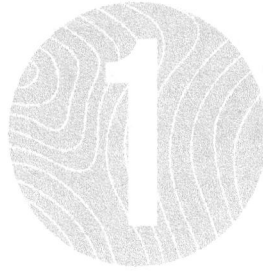

GROUNDED GREATNESS: DANCE WITH THE EARTH

"To touch the earth is to have harmony with nature."
— **Oglala Lakota Proverb.**

Journey into Rio Secreto

We had planned a grand family reunion in Cancun, a sun-soaked paradise where fun meets relaxation. Yet, as the trip neared, our gathering of 20 dwindled to just the four of us: myself, my wife, and our two boys. While I'm not one to lounge poolside at a resort, a bit of sun-soaked stillness can be appealing. But with our crowd reduced, I dug deeper, hunting for an adventure that whispered more than ocean breezes and margaritas. That's when I stumbled upon Rio Secreto.

Rio Secreto, an underground river winding through breathtaking caves, is a testament to Mexico's ancient marvels. In Mayan culture, these caves held a sacred space, a hidden world where water, silence, and time converge. Diving into its depths would be a richer experience than lazing by the pool.

Upon arrival, we were briefed: no phones, no chatter. Just Mother Earth in her most primal form. Adorned in wetsuits and headlights, we descended single file into this underworld. The caves shrouded us in complete darkness, filled only by the sound of cool, serene water sweeping past us. The water crept higher, from our ankles to our waists, rising to neck level, until suddenly, it enveloped us in depths exceeding 20 feet. There we were, over 100 feet below the surface, surrounded by stillness profound enough to blur not just the lines of sight but the borders of the self. Where did my body end? Where did the Earth begin? For a moment, we were seamless.

At one point, we switched off our headlights and sank into silence. For five whole minutes, absolute darkness and silence engaged us in a meditation like no other, a harmonious union with Earth. Though surrounded by Cancun's bustling tourist trap, there was a profound connection: life meeting life.

Emerging from the caves, the transformation lingered. Breathing felt lighter, my heart calmer, and heart rate variability surged, gently affirming my body's relaxed, parasympathetic state. My very being sought this primal reconnection, a communion of life lost amidst modern chaos.

Connection with Earth

Picture yourself standing barefoot on the earth, no shoes, no barriers, just you and the ground beneath your feet. It's not just dirt. It's a living, breathing force. Every blade of grass, every grain of soil, every pulse of energy beneath you is part of a story far older than civilization itself. And here's the truth as ancient as humanity:

We rise from the Earth and, inevitably, return to it.

I learned this firsthand as a child, running wild through the untamed landscapes of Africa. My father's work with the United Nations and the World Bank brought us to places where modern convenience had not yet severed the bond between humans and the land. I watched the Hadzabe tribe move through the bush with effortless grace, their bare feet molding to the terrain like an old handshake between body and earth. They weren't thinking about "grounding" or "negative ions" or "microbiomes." They were simply living *in rhythm, in connection, in sync.*

Flash forward a few decades, and I'm in a radiology suite, staring at MRI scans of degenerated spines, misaligned joints, and bodies riddled with inflammation. The human frame, designed to thrive in nature, is now trapped in ergonomic chairs and cushioned soles and is slowly losing its primal intelligence. As a physician, I see the consequences of this disconnect daily. As a descendant of woodworkers, I understand that the material matters; whether it's the grain of a tree or the bones of a body, structure and function are inseparable. Ancient wisdom has been whispering this truth for centuries: **We are designed to move with the earth, not against it.** Somewhere along the way, we stopped listening.

We replaced dirt paths with concrete sidewalks, sunrise walks with screen time, and the healing touch of nature with the numbing hum of modern life. But here's the good news: We can reclaim what's been lost. We can step out of our cushioned cages and rediscover what our ancestors knew in their bones.

In this chapter, we'll explore the science behind that primal connection, how walking barefoot strengthens more than just your feet, how the soil beneath you is teeming with life that your gut needs, and why plunging into cold water can reboot your nervous system like a factory reset. We'll dive into forest bathing, circadian rhythms, and the underestimated power of standing in the sun.

The Earth isn't just where we come from. It's where we heal. So, let's get our hands (and feet) dirty. It's time to dance with the Earth again.

Harnessing the Power of Grounding

The simple act of connecting skin to the soil, known as grounding or earthing, is as ancient as humanity. Our ancestors were rooted to the earth for millennia. However, modern life has broken this primal bond. Science now suggests that reconnecting with the planet may do more than soothe the soul; it might also be a potent ally in reducing inflammation and enhancing immune function.

At its core, grounding revolves around the idea that direct contact with the earth allows the transfer of electrons from the ground into the body. The Earth's surface carries a subtle negative charge, which can potentially neutralize free radicals and reduce oxidative stress in the body. One major contributor to chronic disease is persistent inflammation, often driven by an overload of free radicals. This theory proposes that by absorbing free electrons from the earth, grounding can combat free radical damage and thus, inflammation.

Several studies have explored the physiological impacts of grounding, especially its potential to mitigate inflammation. Researchers have examined the effects of grounding on inflammation markers. Subjects in small sample studies who slept on grounded conductive mats were found to have reduced levels of inflammation-related biomarkers, such as cortisol, indicating diminished stress responses. The experiment demonstrated that grounded subjects also had normalized circadian cortisol profiles, suggesting improved stress recovery and inflammation control.

Moreover, other similar studies have found that grounding could influence immune responses. Participants who were grounded exhibited lower white blood cell counts and reduced pain, swelling, and redness at injury sites, indicating that grounding may potentially dampen the inflammatory response by modulating the immune system.

Grounding anchors us back to the Earth, rekindling an ancient bond essential for our health and equilibrium. Research suggests that these simple connections with the ground beneath our feet could provide solutions to modern health issues by reducing inflammation, boosting immunity, and fostering a sense of well-being.

As we journey through this book, we will implement grounding, not just an act but as a return home, a simple yet profound step toward lifelong vitality.

Barefoot Brilliance: Walking Your Way to Strength, Balance, and Brainpower

Walking barefoot on the earth invites a healing journey, a seemingly simple practice with profound effects. It's a neurological, muscular, and evolutionary reset. The human foot is a remarkable example of form and function: 26 bones, 33 joints, over 100 muscles, and thousands of nerve endings, all orchestrating movement and balance. The moment you ditch your shoes, you activate an entire sensory system masked by modern footwear.

It all comes down to proprioception, your body's internal GPS. This system, which means "one's own perception," relies on mechanoreceptors in your skin, muscles, and joints to constantly update your brain about where you are in space. The more feedback your feet provide, the sharper your balance, coordination, and agility become.

Studies show that walking barefoot increases proprioceptive input, enhances motor control, and reduces fall risk, which is especially crucial as we age. However, a barefoot lifestyle is not just about foot health; it is brain training disguised as movement.

Think of modern shoes as a cast, it's supportive but it engenders weakness over time. With every step in thick soles, the small stabilizing muscles of your feet get lazier. Walk barefoot, and suddenly, those neglected muscles, tendons, and ligaments start pulling their weight.

Research shows that barefoot walking and minimalist footwear significantly activate intrinsic foot muscles, improving posture, gait, and overall functional movement. It's natural strength training; no gym membership is required.

Sensory feedback from the ground helps with balance, stimulates neural pathways, and strengthens the brain's ability to process movement. Studies have found that barefoot walking improves reaction time, spatial awareness, and cognitive resilience. And for our city-dwelling friends with concrete jungles underfoot, there's no need to miss out! Explore conductive barefoot-type shoes. These nifty innovations offer the natural feel and mobility of barefoot walking while keeping you connected with the earth, providing a touch of rural benefits in urban settings.

The takeaway? Your feet are meant to move, feel, and adapt, not to be trapped in a lifetime of rubber insulation. Every barefoot step is a return to nature, a strength-building exercise, and a neurological boost.

Tracing the Evolution of the Human Foot: A Radiologist's Insight

Get ready to take a step back in time as we uncover the fascinating evolution of the human foot, from our barefoot ancestors' to today's often-shoe-bound generation's. In my work as a radiologist, diving into foot anatomy reveals more than just bone structures; it unveils tales of change driven by culture, lifestyle, and technology.

Modern shoes have wrapped, cushioned, and constrained our feet in ways that contrast with the natural conditions under which human feet evolved. The result? Subtle yet significant changes in foot anatomy and biomechanics are reflected in the X-rays and MRIs examined in my department.

Weakened Foot Muscles

Imagine your feet working like a top-notch orchestra; each muscle, tendon, and ligament plays its part in a symphony of movement and support. Yet, modern footwear, with its plush cushioning and supportive arches, leaves these muscles lounging in the green room. Over time, this can lead to weaker muscles and compromised stability.

Reduced Sensory Feedback

Barefoot walking amplifies proprioception, the body's ability to sense its location in space and movement. Cushioned soles, while comforting, create a barrier to this feedback. It's akin to dancing in earmuffs; you lose the nuances that guide balance and posture.

Altered Foot Shape

Ah, the narrow-toe box! Fashion demands neat lines, but at what cost? Radiology reveals how toes, previously splayed in barefoot populations, have been nudged together into bunion-producing bundles, transforming natural toe alignment over time.

Arch Changes

Our feet thrive on engagement, with their arches acting as built-in shock absorbers. But when shoes do the lifting, these arches relax, weakening over time. From an X-ray perspective, you can see the flat-foot syndrome playing out; it's a common modern malady in a world obsessed with support.

Altered Gait Mechanics

Modern footwear, particularly those with raised heels, encourages a heel-strike walking pattern that changes gait mechanics. This creates higher impact forces affecting knees and hips. In stark contrast, barefoot walking leads to a more forefoot stride, better distributing these forces across joints.

Radiology: A Time Capsule for Foot Evolution

When comparing ancient and modern foot anatomy through radiological imaging, the discrepancies are apparent:

1. **Arch Structure:**
   - Ancient Foot: Stronger arches, as seen in radiographs, indicated by well-aligned bones like the navicular and cuboid.
   - Modern Foot: Flattened arches or evident arch support reliance, often revealed through increased plantar fascia thickness.

2. **Toe Alignment:**
   - Ancient Foot: Naturally spread toes, aligned with metatarsophalangeal joints.
   - Modern Foot: Frequent display of bunions and hammertoes, with visible misalignment and joint deformities.

3. Bone Density:

- Ancient Foot: Greater bone density due to challenging, uneven terrains promoting bone health.
- Modern Foot: Reduced bone density, with a tendency towards osteoporosis in older populations.

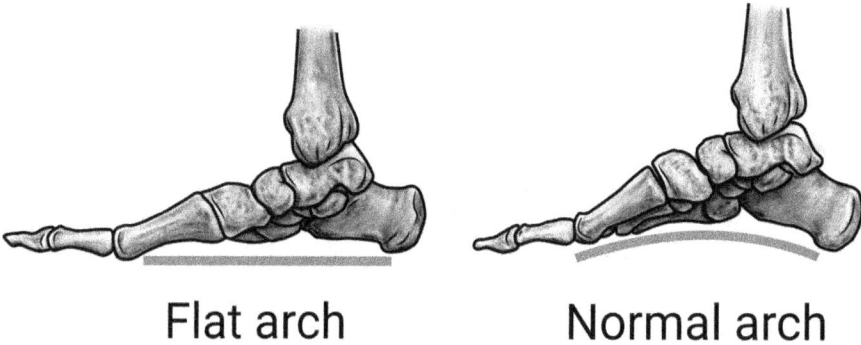

Flat arch   Normal arch

The Barefoot Reawakening

Today's footwear has caused anatomical shifts, as seen in radiology images. Soft padding and constrained space have caused comprehensive structural modifications, resulting in weakened muscles, altered arches, and changed foot mechanics.

Research illustrates that modern footwear has increased the incidence of conditions such as plantar fasciitis and bunions, resulting from compromised natural movement. Barefoot populations, on the other hand, show fewer foot-related ailments and maintain a natural strength and alignment we can appreciate from a radiological standpoint.

Consider incorporating more barefoot activities or minimalist footwear to restore natural foot function and structure and promote foot health. Barefoot activities enhance muscular engagement, foster proper arch support, and lead to healthier overall gait patterns.

Understanding the radiological and anatomical differences between ancient and modern feet reminds us of footwear's profound impact on our natural biomechanics, a lesson, quite literally, underfoot.

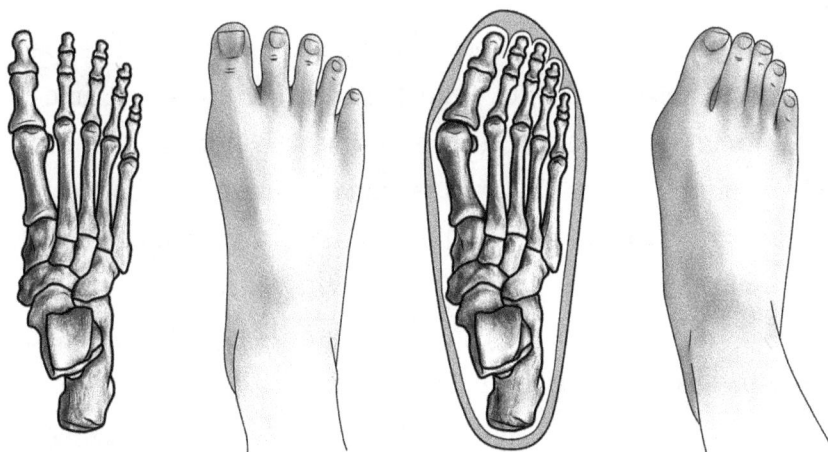

Natural foot shape

Long term effects
of tapered shoes

The Transformative Power of Green Therapy

The Art of Shinrin-Yoku

As we feel the earth beneath our bare feet, reconnecting with our primal instincts and awakening our body's awareness, let us journey deeper into nature's abode. In this place, the tranquility of the forest calls our attention to restoration. Enter the practice of forest bathing, or shinrin-yoku. This Japanese tradition invites us to expose ourselves to the forest's secret healing qualities, which stem from its organic landscapes and health-promoting scents. This practice offers numerous mental and physical health benefits.

Emerging from Japan in the 1980s, the concept of shinrin-yoku, or "forest bathing," invites one to step into the healing sanctuary of the woods—no towels or soap required! It's about immersing ourselves in the forest atmosphere, allowing life to communicate with life and creating an intimate bridge between nature and well-being. This simple yet profound practice enables participants to connect deeply with nature's healing powers, nurturing mental clarity and emotional balance.

Scientific evidence supports forest bathing as a remarkable experience and highlights its numerous benefits. Studies show that spending time in wooded areas can dramatically reduce cortisol levels, the notorious stress hormone, effectively calming the body's stress response. When surrounded by towering trees and lush green foliage, individuals frequently report lower blood pressure, reduced muscle tension, and a profound inner peace. Our connection to the earth nurtures the mind and body in ways science only begins to understand.

Beyond the visual artistry of majestic trees and filtered light, forests offer a vibrant symphony of nature's sounds: the rhythmic rustle and bustle of leaves moving in the wind and the melodic calls of various birds. This healing ambiance creates a soothing harmony that calms the mind, lowers the brain's fight-or-flight response, boosts mood, and enhances overall psychological well-being.

Beyond this naturescape are health-promoting phytoncides, natural aromatic compounds that trees secrete to ward off pests and pathogens. Think of them as nature's aromatherapy. As you breathe in the forest air, you inhale these phytoncides, which studies have shown to enhance human natural killer (NK) cell activity. This immune boost strengthens your body's defenses, making you more resilient to illness. The forest is a multisensory experience that harmonizes with your biology to enhance health, uplift mood, and foster a deeper connection between the individual and nature.

Incorporating forest bathing into your routine is the green prescription for holistic health. This is not about completing your daily steps but allowing the forest to engage all your senses. Feel the texture of the bark, inhale the rich aromatic compounds, and let your eyes shift through the shades of green.

Research shows that spending as little as 15 minutes in a natural setting can significantly lower cortisol levels, reduce heart rate, and improve overall mood. This aligns with findings that natural exposure stimulates parasympathetic nervous system activity, promoting relaxation and recovery, essential for health and longevity. In contrast to fast-paced modern life, the forest remains calm and steadfast, beckoning us to hit reset.

Nature Immersion to Ion Infusion

Just as shinrin-yoku, or forest bathing, reconnects us with the natural world, let us now explore how the air we breathe in these environments enhances our health. Imagine walking near a waterfall or through a dense forest. The air feels crisper and fresher. It is not just your imagination; it is science at play. Waterfalls, forests, and oceans emit an abundance of negative ions. These invisible molecules come bursting forth when air molecules are broken apart by sunlight, radiation, or moving air and water.

These negative ions, far from being bad news despite their name, enhance air quality and benefit respiratory function and mental clarity. Think of them as the air's equivalent of a natural power-up; they cling to positively charged particles like dust, pollen, and pollutants, effectively neutralizing and purifying the air. Exposure to negative ions may also reduce inflammation.

Research is developing on how environments rich in negative ions can influence our health. Exposure to negative air ions can affect the c-fos gene's expression (a neuronal activity marker) and regulate serotonin levels. This regulation may influence mood and overall well-being. Meanwhile, other studies have noted that negative ions improve respiratory function, as they help clear airways and bolster lung capacity by reducing airborne irritants. It is as if the very atmosphere of these natural settings sings to our physiology, enabling us to breathe easier, think more clearly, and feel more relaxed, all tangible gifts from nature's laboratory.

Beyond just clearing the air we breathe, negative ions create an inviting embrace of well-being. These natural settings stimulate parasympathetic nervous system activity, inducing a state of relaxation, and in some cultures, are considered sanctuaries for spiritual refreshment. Historically, people have flocked to waterfalls, seashores, and expansive forests for scenic views and the unseen health benefits delivered through their natural air purification powers.

Healing in the Wild: Ecotherapy & Cognitive Health

In our increasingly digital world, filled with constant notifications and information overload, it has become easy to forget the profound benefits of spending time in nature. As a neuroradiologist, my work revolves around analyzing intricate brain images, understanding the complexities of cognitive health, and witnessing firsthand how our physical and emotional environments affect our well-being. The more I delve into my profession, the clearer it becomes:

Nature isn't just a pretty backdrop; it's an essential ingredient for optimal brain function and cognitive vitality.

Research has established a compelling connection between exposure to natural environments and mental health improvement. Studies have shown that spending time in green spaces can significantly reduce cortisol levels, the stress hormone negatively impacting cognitive performance and emotional well-being. When cortisol levels drop, the brain is free to function at its best.

Moreover, contact with nature and subsequent stress reduction can support more optimal brain-derived neurotrophic factor (BDNF) levels, a protein crucial for the growth and survival of neurons. Higher BDNF levels enhance neuroplasticity, allowing the brain to adapt, reorganize, and rejuvenate itself in the face of aging or injury. Immersing ourselves in nature invigorates our neural pathways and nurtures our cognitive resources, creating a healthier mindset and sharper memory. Strolling through a park or hiking in the woods can create significant neurochemical shifts within the brain, promoting clarity, relaxation, and creativity.

Eco-therapy is nature's way of healing the mind, offering psychological boosts as grounded in science as they are in the earth itself. The sights, sounds, and even the feel of nature engage our senses, making eco-therapy a holistic tune-up for our primal connections. It clears the mind and brings emotional balance. Spending time in nature boosts cognitive function and sparks creativity while dialing down the amygdala's stress response. So, a stroll through the woods is not just a break from work but a brain boost.

When immersed in a natural setting, you engage in what ecopsychologists call "soft fascination," effortless attention that allows the brain to recover from the relentless demands of directed focus (called "hard fascination"). Researchers find that taking it easy in nature recharges our mental batteries and provides restorative effects on cognitive functioning.

Learning Resilience from Biodiversity

As we stroll through the healing embrace of eco-therapy, the natural world beckons us to explore the vibrant tapestry of biodiversity. Just as a garden with diverse plants blooms more robustly, humans flourish better in multifaceted environments. Biodiversity is not just a fancy ecological term, it is the cornerstone of mental resilience and well-being.

Diving into the richness of biodiverse settings exposes us to a symphony of stimuli, each subtly fine-tuning our mental health. These environments are not merely bustling with plants and animals; they vibrate with diverse sounds, textures, and colors that engage our minds in an all-encompassing sensory dance. Research reveals that hanging out in biodiverse spaces bolsters psychological resilience and combats urban stress. In short, the richer the biodiversity, the greater the therapeutic punch, providing a natural shield against the stresses of city life.

Biodiversity teaches us resilience through its complex web of life. Each biome thrives on adaptability, showcasing intricate interconnections similar to our societal relationships. By nurturing environments that house many species, we invite lessons in resilience and diversity into our lives. Individuals exposed to diverse natural settings exhibit better emotional resilience and cognitive flexibility, crucial traits for navigating life's twists and turns. Our inherent draw to serene, biodiverse landscapes may be because they quietly coach us in finding balance and enduring challenges.

With their concrete facades and relentless pace, cities often lack nature's complexity, leading to sensory dullness and mental weariness. By weaving biodiversity pockets like lush parks and communal gardens into urban landscapes, cities can emulate the restful benefits of more pristine natural settings. Implementing biophilic design, focusing on reconnecting humans with nature, can transform downtowns into lush sanctuaries, inviting moments of peace amid the chaos. As we embrace biodiversity, we tap into nature's wisdom, learning resilience through variety and interdependence. Each element contributes to a harmonious whole, offering insights into adaptation and balance that echo throughout life's journey.

The Wisdom of Trees: A Woodworker's Perspective on Nature's Healers

I grew up surrounded by wood, the scent of freshly cut timber, the feel of grain under my fingertips, the quiet dignity of a fallen tree reborn as furniture. My family's woodworking tradition wasn't just about craftsmanship, it was about respect. We never cut down trees unnecessarily. Instead, we salvaged old, fallen wood, breathing new life into what nature had already given. Every slab of wood told a story of storms weathered, years counted in rings, and beauty that deepened with age.

It still fascinates me that many trees live for centuries, quietly witnessing history unfold beneath their branches. Some have stood since before the Industrial Revolution, before our modern diseases, and before the rise and fall of entire civilizations. Methuselah, the 4,853-year-old bristlecone pine in California's White Mountains, has seen more history than any of us ever will, and will likely outlive us too.

Science is now catching up to what ancient cultures have long understood: **Being around trees is aesthetically pleasing and biologically healing.**

But trees are not just compassionate providers of shade and oxygen; they are part of an intricate, intelligent network. Forests operate as a collective. Trees communicate through underground fungal networks, sometimes called the "wood wide web." They send chemical signals through their roots, warning each other of pests or droughts. When one tree is cut down, neighboring trees detect the distress and respond biologically, adjusting their growth, fortifying themselves, and even sharing nutrients. There's a lesson here. Trees survive not through isolation but through interdependence. They thrive as a community, supporting one another through unseen connections.

Apart from the well-documented health benefits of green therapy, we also have something deeper to learn from trees: unity, resilience, and the power of collective strength. In a world that often pushes independence as the ultimate virtue, trees hold a different kind of wisdom that reminds us we are stronger together.

So, the next time you pass an ancient oak or a towering pine, take a moment to feel the presence of something older, wiser, and deeply connected. The trees were here long before us; if we allow them to, they might teach us how to live.

Earth's Embrace: An Indian Heritage of Harmony

In the ancient wisdom of India, Earth (Prithvi) is not just soil beneath our feet; it is the mother, the foundation, the silent witness to our existence. It nourishes, stabilizes, and ultimately reclaims us when our time is done. In yoga and Ayurveda, and from our primal health perspective, the Earth element is more than a metaphor; it is the very fabric of our being.

In Indian heritage, the reverence for soil and earth is intricately woven into cultural practices, reflecting a deep understanding of our place in the universe. Yet, in the modern world, we have lost this connection. We walk on concrete instead of soil, sleep indoors disconnected from Earth's grounding force, and toil away in artificial lighting instead of natural daylight. But in the wisdom of Ayurveda, yoga, and the Pancha Bhutas (the five primal elements), the Earth is not a mere resource. It is sacred intelligence that forms and dissolves life.

The Pancha Bhutas: The Five Elements of Existence

"Pancha Bhutas" is a Sanskrit term referring to the five elements of nature: Prithvi (earth), Jal (water), Agni (fire), Vayu (air), and Akasha (space). These elements are venerated as the fundamental building blocks of life. Earth is regarded as the most foundational, serving as the bedrock upon which all life flourishes.

Ancient Indian thought sees the human body as being composed of the five primal elements:

1. **Prithvi (Earth):** The bones, muscles, and tissues—our structure, stability, and physical form.

2. **Jal (Water):** The blood, lymph, plasma—fluidity, nourishment, and flow.

3. **Agni (Fire):** The metabolism, digestion, and inner radiance—the force of transformation.

4. **Vayu (Air):** The breath, nervous system, and circulation—movement and life force.

5. **Akasha (Space):** The emptiness within cells, the pause between breaths—expansion and potential.

This is not poetry. This is primal biology articulated thousands of years ago. Every function of our body is an interplay of these forces. When they are balanced, we thrive. When disrupted, disease takes hold.

No ancient tradition embodies the Pancha Bhutas more profoundly than cremation. In India, death is a sacred dissolution, a return of the borrowed elements to their source. This isn't just religious belief, it is biological reality. The body is a loan from nature, and the moment we stop clinging to it, we align with the wisdom of the cosmos.

Modern culture fears death, but ancient traditions embraced it as a return home. By honoring the Pancha Bhutas, we don't just live well, we learn how to die well, too.

Prithvi in Yoga: The Root of Stability

Ancient yoga is not just movement, it is alignment with the elemental forces. Prithvi is related to the Muladhara (Root Chakra), the energy center at the base of the spine. The Muladhara governs our sense of stability, survival, and connection to the physical world. A weak Muladhara leads to anxiety, instability, and physical frailty, modern ailments of the disconnected human.

Primal yogic practices that **restore the Earth element** include:

Walking barefoot (Earthing): As we discussed, it reduces inflammation and balances cortisol levels.

Sitting on the ground: A forgotten practice that improves posture, digestion, and spinal alignment.

Grounding meditations: Visualizing deep roots anchoring into the Earth to cultivate stability and resilience.

Modern life pulls us off the ground, literally and metaphorically. But the wisdom of yoga reminds us that **when we return to the Earth, we return to ourselves.**

Prithvi is not just soil but memory, stability, and life itself. To reclaim health, longevity, and peace, we must return to the wisdom beneath our feet.

Science of Cold: Unlocking the Primal Code of Resilience

Long before heated homes and Gore-Tex jackets, our ancestors faced the raw, untamed elements daily. Winter wasn't a season to be avoided; it was a crucible that forged resilience. Cold wasn't just endured. It was a physiological call to arms, activating primal survival mechanisms that modern comfort has lulled into dormancy. Enter cold immersion and thermogenesis, not as wellness fads, but as the rekindling of ancient biological intelligence.

Cold immersion offers multiple health benefits including improved circulation. When you step into a chilly stream or take a bracing dip in a cold lake, your body goes into a controlled shock. Vasoconstriction occurs, driving blood away from your extremities to protect vital organs. Once you emerge from the water, your body works double-time to reheat itself, improving circulation.

Research suggests that this kind of temperature oscillation enhances vascular tone and encourages better blood flow through capillaries. Do not be surprised if you feel like you have just received a high-octane dose of energy after a brief swim in cold waters because your body's inner furnace is now working at peak efficiency.

Then, there is the undeniable mood boost. Cold immersion is known for ramping up endorphins, the body's natural "feel-good" chemicals. These chemicals not only mitigate pain but also elevate your spirits. Studies found that cold water swimming significantly improved the mood of participants, who reported increased energy and reduced tension, fatigue, and depression.

Cold exposure triggers a cascade of responses that sharpen the body's adaptability, turning sluggish metabolic pathways into high-performance engines. At the heart of this process is non-shivering thermogenesis (NST), where the body generates heat without the violent muscle contractions of shivering. The key player?

Brown Adipose Tissue (BAT) – This metabolically active fat burns energy instead of storing it, releasing heat. Unlike the inert white fat accumulating from excess calories, BAT is a primal fuel furnace linked to improved insulin sensitivity, fat oxidation, and longevity.

But the benefits of cold immersion go beyond burning fat. Cold is a classic example of **hormesis**, a biological principle where small, controlled stressors strengthen the body. Exposure to cold water or icy air flips powerful switches in the nervous system:

> **Noradrenaline Surge** – A cold plunge can spike noradrenaline, sharpen focus, boost mood, and enhance cognitive resilience.

> **Dopamine Elevation** – Cold immersion causes a sustained rise in dopamine, which creates a lasting feeling of alertness, motivation, and well-being. This is a natural antidepressant effect.

> **Mitochondrial Biogenesis** – Cold forces cells to build more mitochondria, increasing energy efficiency and metabolic flexibility.

Autophagy Activation – Brief cold stress triggers cellular cleanup, breaking down damaged proteins and renewing tissues at a molecular level.

Our ancestors didn't need cryotherapy chambers; they had rivers, oceans, and snow. The Wim Hofs of the Paleolithic world weren't anomalies; they were the norm. Those who adapted to the cold survived, thrived, and evolved.

Cold immersion reconnects us with this primal challenge, reawakening dormant survival circuitry that modernity has numbed. That's why cold plunges feel like a visceral physical, mental, and emotional reboot. The shock of cold isn't just temperature; it's an ancient signal telling the body, *"Wake up. Adapt. Overcome."*

At its core, aging is a loss of metabolic flexibility and cellular resilience. Cold exposure reverses this trend, training the body to endure, adapt, and regenerate. The modern world has given us comfort but at the cost of resilience.

If you are wondering whether braving the cold is just about some physiological amusement, it is not. This practice taps into ancient resilience, hinting at our evolutionary history and our capacity to thrive in diverse, sometimes extreme, climates. It reminds us, like the soil beneath our feet, that our bodies and minds are poised to push boundaries, embrace challenges, and grow stronger.

Cold isn't the enemy. It's a forgotten partner. Embrace it and reclaim your primal resilience.

Cold Showers to Circadian Clocks

Just as the icy embrace of water renews the spirit, sunlight's golden rays play an instrumental role in tuning our internal clocks and revitalizing our energy levels. The sun does not just fuel photosynthesis; it is the maestro governing sleep-wake cycles and hormone release. Humans are hardwired to follow the sun's cues, marking the time since our sunbaked ancestors first roamed the earth. Regular exposure to natural light is crucial for aligning this internal clock, making daylight more essential than your morning coffee.

Once upon a time, before alarm clocks jolted us into consciousness and LED screens bathed us in artificial twilight, our biology danced to the rhythm of the cosmos. The sun was our timekeeper, the night our sanctuary. But we've declared war on this ancient synchronization in the modern world. We binge-watch past midnight, wake up to the grating buzz of an alarm, drown ourselves in caffeine, and wonder why we feel perpetually exhausted, inflamed, and metabolically broken. The answer? We've severed our connection with the most primal force of all: **circadian rhythm**, the biological master clock that governs every cell in our body.

A well-synchronized circadian rhythm affects everything from when we feel sleepy to the peak of our alertness. This rhythm is regulated by exposure to natural light, which suppresses melatonin, the hormone that whispers sleepiness to our bodies as darkness falls. Exposure to bright morning light improves sleep patterns and increases overall alertness. Think of natural light as the nudge your internal metronome needs to keep perfect time. Workers exposed to natural light in their office environments showed significantly improved mood and productivity compared to those toiling under artificial lights.

At its core, circadian rhythm is a 24-hour biological cycle encoded deep within our DNA. All systems (metabolism, immunity, cognition, and mood) align with the sun's movement. When we honor this rhythm, we thrive. When we disrupt it, disease sets in. Research on the molecular mechanisms of circadian rhythm, which demonstrated that our biological clocks regulate gene expression, metabolism, and longevity, earned the Nobel Prize in Physiology and Medicine in 2017.

Yet modern life throws our circadian machinery into chaos. Artificial light, late-night eating, shift work, and excessive screen exposure send mixed signals, forcing our bodies into a biological jet lag, a chronic mismatch between internal time and external reality.

The Science of Circadian Disruption

Metabolic Breakdown: Eating out of sync with the sun impairs insulin sensitivity, increasing the risk of obesity, type 2 diabetes, and metabolic syndrome. Nighttime snacking is a bad idea. The body is metabolically primed to process food during daylight. Late-night eating leads to fat accumulation, poor glucose control, and digestive dysfunction.

Cognitive & Mood Decline: Blue light exposure after sunset suppresses melatonin production, delaying sleep onset and impairing brain detoxification, memory consolidation, and mood regulation. Chronic circadian misalignment is linked to depression, anxiety, and neurodegenerative diseases like Alzheimer's.

Immune System Dysfunction & Inflammation: Circadian disruption weakens immune responses, increasing susceptibility to infections, autoimmune diseases, and cancer. Night shift workers experience chronic inflammation and a higher risk of cardiovascular disease.

The Primal Health Blueprint: How to Resync with Your Circadian Clock

The good news? Recalibrating your circadian rhythm requires primal intelligence, not a time machine.

1. Chase the Sun (Morning Sunlight = Circadian Anchor)
- Sunlight before 10 a.m. triggers a morning cortisol pulse, signaling wakefulness and priming metabolism.
- 20–30 minutes of natural light exposure enhances mood, focus, and sleep quality.

2. Dim the Lights, Respect the Dark
- Ditch blue light after sunset; use red bulbs, candlelight, or blue-light-blocking glasses.
- Early to bed, early to rise; your genes expect darkness by 10

p.m. for optimal melatonin secretion.

3. Time-Restricted Eating: Eat in Sync with Your Biology

- Align meals with the sun. Consume calories within a 6-to 10-hour window, ideally from morning to early evening.
- Fasting at night optimizes cellular repair (autophagy), digestion, and metabolism.

4. Move with the Light, Rest with the Dark

- Exercise in daylight to sync metabolic cycles and enhance sleep quality.
- Avoid high-intensity workouts close to bedtime, as they can spike cortisol and disrupt sleep.

Circadian Alignment = Longevity & Resilience

Our ancestors didn't check their phones at 2 a.m. or eat midnight snacks under fluorescent lights. They woke with the sun, ate when the light was strong, and rested when darkness fell. Their biology worked because they lived in alignment with nature's clock.

The modern world has pulled us out of sync, but the solution isn't complicated. It's a return to primal intelligence. A simple shift in light exposure, meal timing, and sleep habits can restore our health, boost energy, and even slow biological aging.

Circadian rhythm isn't just a wellness trend, it's the ancient programming of life itself. Honor it, and you honor your health.

Earthbound Vitality:
Reconnecting for Healing and Harmony

As we conclude this chapter, let us anchor ourselves in the profound truth that we come from the Earth and will eventually return to it. The Earth is not merely a backdrop to our existence but an active partner in our well-being, one that nourishes, heals, and restores us when we intentionally engage with it.

Grounding, our physical connection with the Earth, recharges and vitalizes us subtly and profoundly. Our primal design is intricately engineered to interact with this planet, as evidenced by the remarkable mechanics of our feet, designed to sense, stabilize, and connect with the ground beneath us.

The forest, teeming with life and rich in ionized air, is not just a sanctuary for the mind but also a dynamic healing space for the body. Brimming with microbial biodiversity, the soil forms a foundation for our internal ecosystem, shaping immunity, digestion, and mental clarity.

The Earth's day and night cycles are more than time markers; they prime our circadian rhythms and align us with our biological design. When we lose touch with these natural cycles, we lose touch with the rhythm of life itself.

And finally, the immense biodiversity of the Earth—plants, fungi, animals, and even the tiniest microbes—offers us an unparalleled reservoir of healing resources. The ecosystems that sustain life remind us of the interwoven fabric of existence:

Our health reflects the Earth's health.

In ancient Indian philosophy, the Earth, or Prithvi, was revered as a sacred mother, a living entity imbued with nurturing and healing powers. The Vedas, some of the oldest spiritual texts in human history, describe Prithvi as a life-giving force, a source of stability and abundance. This reverence extended to the soil, rivers, mountains, and forests, all seen as extensions of her divine essence. Ancient practices such as yoga and Ayurveda emphasized harmony with Prithvi, recognizing that our physical and spiritual well-being are inextricably tied to the health of the Earth. By honoring Prithvi, we embrace a timeless wisdom that reminds us to treat the Earth not as a resource to exploit, but as a healer to revere.

To the Hadzabe, the Earth is not merely a place they inhabit but a living, sacred entity that sustains their entire way of life. Every aspect of their existence (food, shelter, medicine, and even their sense of community) is deeply rooted in their connection to the land.

The Hadzabe move through their environment with respect and mindfulness, taking only what they need and giving thanks for what the Earth provides. Their intimate knowledge of the flora and fauna and reliance on natural cycles reflect a deep trust in the Earth as a provider and healer. For the Hadzabe, the Earth is not a resource to be controlled but a partner to be lived with in harmony, a sentiment that echoes the ancient wisdom found in many cultures, reminding us of the intrinsic bond between humanity and the planet that sustains us.

By reconnecting with the Earth, we return to the essence of our humanity. The deeper this connection, the more vibrant, resilient, and balanced we become. In the design of life, the Earth is not a separate entity. It is a partner, a healer, and a reminder of our origins. Engage with it, and you will rediscover a vitality that no modern intervention can replicate.

Let us take this wisdom forward, honoring our place in this grand, interconnected system. **To thrive is not merely to exist on this Earth but to live in harmony with it.**

Up next, we move inward and tune into the whispers of our bodies.

Primal Practices:

These habits can integrate seamlessly into your daily routine, helping you maintain a balanced connection with the natural world. Incorporating these practices into your routine can improve your balance and strength while fostering a closer connection with your surroundings.

1. Mindful Barefoot Strolls

Carve out a slice of your day to roam barefoot across nature's finest offerings, such as grass, soil, or sand. Known as grounding or earthing, this uncomplicated ritual helps you tap into the Earth's energy, potentially lifting your mood and dissolving stress.

Engage with each step, savoring the unique textures underfoot—a sensory symphony for your feet. As an added perk, this practice primes your foot muscles and boosts proprioception, enhancing your balance and coordination.

Urban dwellers navigating bustling sidewalks can embrace conductive barefoot-type walking shoes that mimic grounding on natural surfaces. These clever creations offer a taste of earthing and the mobility of barefoot walking, keeping your connection to nature alive even amid the high rises.

2. Gardening Gratitude

Spend a few minutes each day tending to a garden, whether an entire backyard plot, a community garden, or simple potted plants on a windowsill. This practice not only relaxes the mind but also exposes you to beneficial microbes in the soil, enhancing your immune system and gut health.

3. Balance-Enhancing Walks

Incorporate balance-focused exercises into your walk routine. Try adding heel-to-toe walking on a straight line, walking backward for short distances, or navigating uneven surfaces like cobblestones or a gentle trail path. These variations challenge your sense of balance and can enhance foot and ankle strength, contributing to overall stability and agility.

4. Immersion in Naturally Ion-Rich Environments

Seek out local parks, forest reserves, or coastlines with waterfalls and lush plant life, and schedule routine visits to soak in the benefits of negative ions. Consider using home ionizers or air purifiers to replicate the beneficial effects of negative ions in your living spaces, particularly in urban environments.

5. Thermoregulation

Cold Showers: Start with 30 seconds at the end of your shower and gradually increase the time. Cold showers invigorate the senses and are a great way to experience increased circulation and a mood boost without needing access to natural bodies of water.

Ice Baths and Cold Plunges: Aim for 2-5 minutes in water around 50°F (10°C) to activate deep thermogenic pathways.

Outdoor Exposure: Ditch the heavy layers in cold weather for short, controlled exposure to natural elements.

Contrast Therapy: Cycle between hot and cold (sauna to cold plunge) to amplify circulation and recovery.

6. Morning Sun Sessions

Aim to spend 20-30 minutes outdoors. Whether sipping your coffee on the porch or walking briskly, basking in morning sunlight can effectively reset your circadian rhythm. Swapping gym visits for outdoor activity rewards your body with movement and light.

7. Biodiversity-Centric Habits

Seek out local reserves or national parks known for their biodiversity and spend weekends or vacations enveloped by nature's complexity. Schedule regular nature-immersion days, prioritizing deep presence in biodiverse surroundings and allowing nature's diverse chorus to guide your reflection.

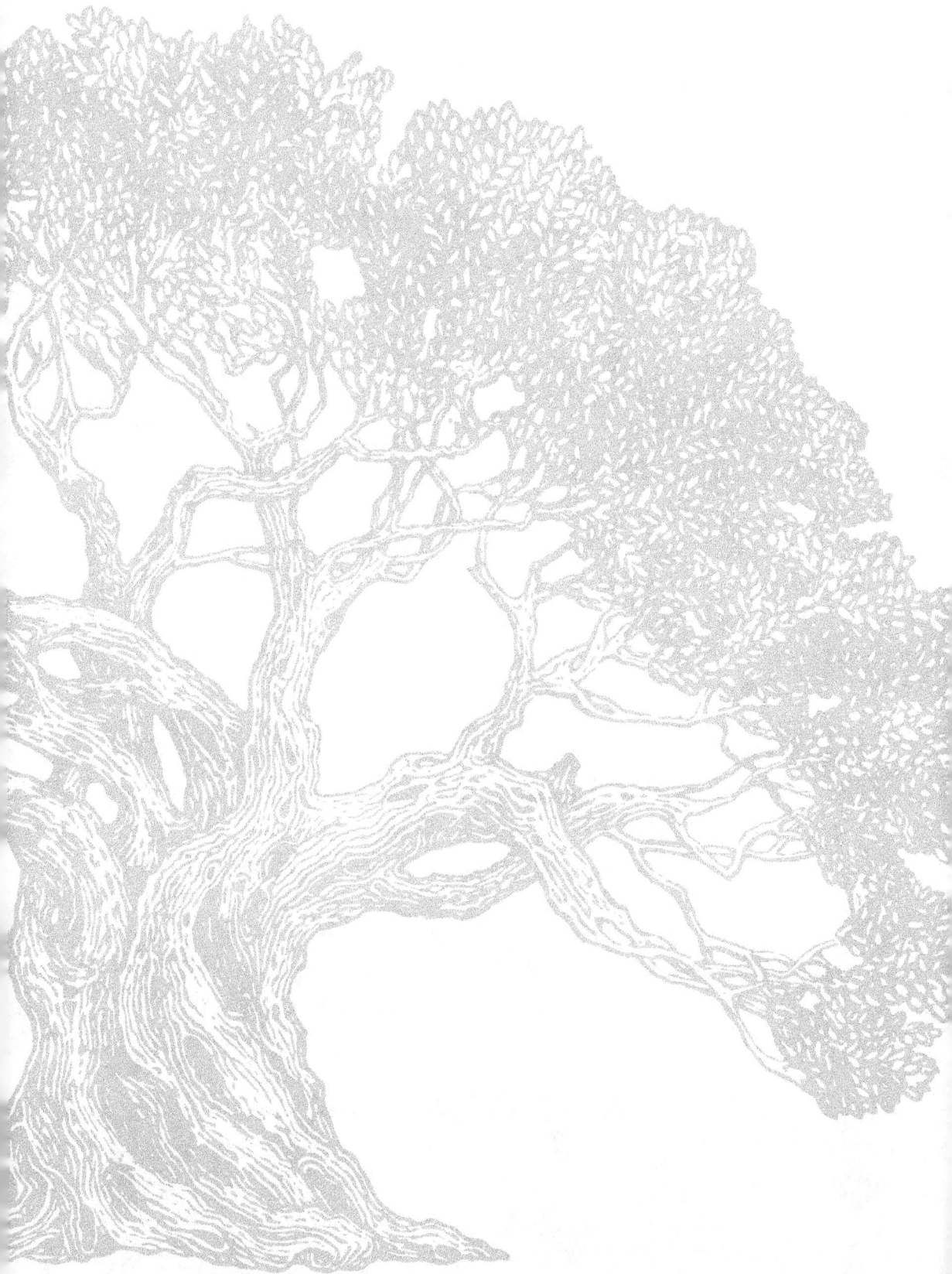

2

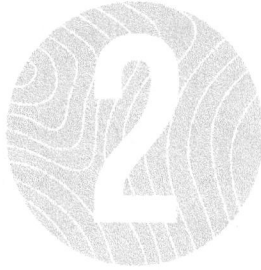

EMBODIED AWARENESS:
EMBRACING THE WISDOM OF OUR BODIES

*"The body is the instrument of our alignment with life;
to ignore its wisdom is to silence the voice of the primal
nature within us."*
– Kavin Mistry, MD

Rediscovering Primal Strength

As a child, watching the Hadzabe engage with their surroundings provided fascinating insights into the raw vitality of human potential. The Hadzabes' lives were integrally linked with balance, endurance, and strength. Daily survival wasn't a theoretical exercise; it was a necessity that built robust bodies capable of incredible stamina, both directly linked to longevity and health. Their hunts weren't measured by modern-day fitness targets like "10,000 steps a day," but instead by the need to traverse vast landscapes in search of nourishment.

Through this journey, I realized that primitive men's true advantage was not merely in the accuracy of an arrow or the weapons they forged but in their bodies' boundless endurance and resilience. These men became masters of the hunt by skill and crafting bodies that could outlast their prey.

Squatting wasn't a workout for the Hadzabe. It was a restful posture that naturally lengthened their spines and grounded them quite literally with the Earth (think ass-to-grass squats for all you gym rats). Since there were no flush toilets in the African savanna, squatting was a regular activity in their lives.

Not only did climbing trees in pursuit of honey provide sweet rewards, but it honed upper and lower body strength, both necessary for survival. Ask a modern city dweller to climb a tree or simply hang from a branch, and you'd be met with skeptical glances or, alas, unfulfilled attempts.

Further, the Hadzabes' resilience, created by carrying weight and walking long distances, enhanced bone density, a guard against osteoporosis. In contrast, my radiology practice frequently reveals the dark side of modernity: osteoporotic hip and vertebral compression fractures, casualties of our increasingly sedentary lifestyles.

Today's modern life, often encapsulated by urban comforts, can lead us away from these primal roots. However, scientific research has been clear: The benefits of maintaining high levels of physical fitness are profound. Measures like VO2 max (the maximum rate at which an individual can consume oxygen during intense exercise) emerge as critical markers for health and longevity. Elevated VO2 max levels are associated with lower risks of cardiovascular diseases, enhanced metabolic health, and improved survival rates.

Moreover, enduring muscle strength, an inherent outcome of a physically active lifestyle, is a pillar of health. Research underscores that greater muscle strength is linked to a lower risk of all-cause mortality, regardless of age or other health conditions. These benefits include decreased risk of falls, enhanced mobility, and improved overall quality of life.

The Hadzabes' lives underscore this fact: Squatting, climbing, and traversing rugged terrain weren't workouts but elements woven into their existence. Their primal living protected them against ailments prevalent in modern societies.

It's time to reignite our body's primal intelligence. We must rediscover that our bodies are engineered for performance, endurance, strength, and flexibility and work toward maximizing these gifts. As we explore this chapter, may we take inspiration from these people who remind us of what we're capable of.

The Geometry of Primal Design

Imagine Leonardo da Vinci's Vitruvian Man stepping off the page as if each of us were a living illustration of nature's affinity for balance and harmony. The human body is a masterpiece of symmetry and geometry, characteristics not only visually striking but crucial for our function and movement.

Our body's design intertwines with mathematics, from the influence of the Fibonacci sequence on our proportions to the Golden Ratio governing our facial structure and even our DNA spirals. This inborn symmetry isn't merely aesthetically pleasing; it plays a vital role in maintaining optimal health and functional harmony.

Consider the alignment of our skeletal structure. Bilateral symmetry (an imaginary vertical line running from head to toe) ensures equal distribution of muscles, bones, and nerves. This symmetry allows for mechanical efficiency, enabling us to walk, run, and dance with precision and grace.

Symmetrical bodies are often healthier and more resilient. Athletes rely on symmetry for enhanced agility and stamina; balanced proportions provide fluidity and reduce the risk of injuries. But what happens when symmetry is disrupted? Deviations from our vertical Y-axis can stress muscles and ligaments, leading to imbalance and discomfort. Symmetry is at the heart of nature's design, a reminder of the elegant balance within us all.

Radiology Reflections on Modern Man

Every day as a radiologist, I have the privilege of peering into the body's internal architecture, the intricate framework that supports us through our daily lives. It's a front-row seat to the silent narrative of how we live, move, and sometimes neglect our bodies. In this role, I've witnessed an intriguing paradox: We are technologically empowered yet physiologically disempowered. In a digital age where information spans the globe at our fingertips, I see the physical form (our bodies) bearing the brunt of modern life's conveniences and misalignments.

This book attempts to raise awareness, from a radiologist's perspective, of the silent decline in human physical empowerment I observe on my screen. As I analyze spine images revealing misalignment, abnormal curvature, or significant endplate degenerative changes, I can't help but wonder: Where did we deviate from the path of vitality? What could we have done to prevent this degeneration? How much is directly linked to our modern, sedentary lifestyles?

The more pressing concern arises when I think about future generations. Today, toddlers are increasingly engaging with technology from day one. What trajectory awaits them if they grow up with habits that inherently disrupt primal alignment and movement? The answers are a bit frightening, and they fuel my determination to discuss these critical issues.

I want to engage active adults, teens, and parents in a conversation that leads to proactive change before we reach irreversible disc degeneration or even herniation. Currently, our approach is lamentably reactive. We wait for symptoms to manifest or a positive imaging finding before attempting to treat the issue. However, considerable damage is done by then, and the root cause remains unaddressed.

The core of the problem is that misalignments and altered biomechanics lead to accelerated degeneration, a pattern I see repeatedly on spine imaging. Initial scans might show instability or minor malalignments, but subsequent images often reveal rapid progression to severe disc degeneration or even herniation. Promoting proper posture and alignment is crucial in preventing this downward spiral, much like maintaining proper tire alignment extends the life of your car's tires.

Think of the body as having a finite tread life, much like Michelin tires. Let's say our knees, shoulders, and hips are designed to last 120 years. What happens when our primal alignment is off? We risk wearing out our joints long before their time, using up the valuable tread life in our 20s and 30s instead of preserving it for an entire lifespan.

That's why a proactive approach is imperative. We must engage in key awareness and preventive measures, assessing and correcting alignment issues upfront. By doing so, we can significantly lengthen the functionality and usability of our human mechanisms. Most disc herniations and joint issues are preventable if only we catch the early signs of instability.

Ultimately, the goal is to prevent you from getting on that treadmill of reactive healthcare. A proactive mindset ensures longevity and vitality, allowing us to thrive in a world that demands more than ever from our bodies. The aim is to foster a healthy, functional body by aligning our modern lives to better reflect our ancestors', whose lives safeguarded survival and cultivated joyous movement.

The Spine: A Pillar of Health

In the ancient yogic tradition, the spine is revered not merely as a structural backbone but as the central channel through which vital energy flows. It is more than just a stack of bones supporting the flesh; it is an architectural marvel that hosts our life force. Spinal alignment is essential for the efficient transfer of loads from feet to head, a seamless blend of stability and mobility. Our body is thus a harmonious, interconnected entity. This holistic perspective sees problems that arise in one area of the body as symptomatic of deeper, systemic imbalances. In essence, there are no isolated joint aches; instead, they often reveal misalignments and disharmonies that resonate throughout the entire being.

Achieving balance and alignment from head to foot isn't just about mirroring elegant postures; it's about establishing a resilient foundation upon which health and longevity depend. The spine mediates this integrative experience, bridging the divide between mindful awareness and physical form. Successful integration requires a willingness to observe and address posture, movement, and alignment throughout the body. By nurturing this holistic perspective, we empower ourselves to identify and rectify imbalances, crafting a system where each part supports the other. As such, emphasizing the health of our spine becomes the cornerstone of comprehensive well-being, allowing the body to thrive in balance and unity.

Among the myriad narratives that unfold in the silent world of medical imaging, skeletal imbalances are one of the most glaring indicators of modern life's toll on the body. At the heart of these imbalances lies the spine. As a radiologist, I frequently witness the jarring reality of this majestic structure burdened by modern habits: reversed cervical curves, thoracic kyphosis (exaggerated curvature) reminiscent of the elderly in much younger patients, and lumbar malalignment whispering the tale of life's silent assaults. When spine alignment deviates, it invites chaos and dysfunction, leading to pain and, ultimately, degeneration.

I've seen extreme cases in my practice, such as complete spinal cord transections due to trauma, rendering patients quadriplegic in an instant. While these are severe scenarios, the reality is that a more commonplace occurrence, such as a disc herniation from years of improper posture, can also be significantly debilitating, interrupting life's harmony and vitality.

Understanding Primal Posture

Posture may seem like a mundane topic, however, it's anything but ordinary. It's the foundational blueprint for our physical health and well-being. Proper human posture is a finely tuned structure designed for optimal balance and efficiency.

Proper posture isn't just about standing tall; it's about how we position our bodies in relation to gravity and our alignment with the ground. This alignment starts at the feet, where each step acts as the first line of defense against the gravitational pull we constantly navigate. When we walk or stand, the weight of our body is transmitted upwards through our feet, ankles, knees, and hips, creating a stable foundation that supports the spine and head.

The ears should align vertically with the shoulders, hips, knees, and ankles to achieve optimal posture. This alignment creates a straight line, distributing body weight evenly and reducing strain on muscles and ligaments. When one component is out of alignment, it can trigger a chain reaction, leading to discomfort, pain, or even injury.

The spine, composed of vertebrae that act as shock absorbers, plays a pivotal role in load transfer. Each section of the spine, the cervical, thoracic, and lumbar, has its natural curvature that absorbs different types of stress while maintaining balance throughout the body. When well-aligned, these curves help distribute weight evenly, minimizing the risk of overloading any single area.

Conversely, improper posture can skew this load transfer, leading to compensatory patterns in the body that can result in chronic pain or other health concerns. For example, if one's head juts forward, it places undue stress on the cervical spine, potentially resulting in tension headaches or neck pain (more on this later).

Types of Posture

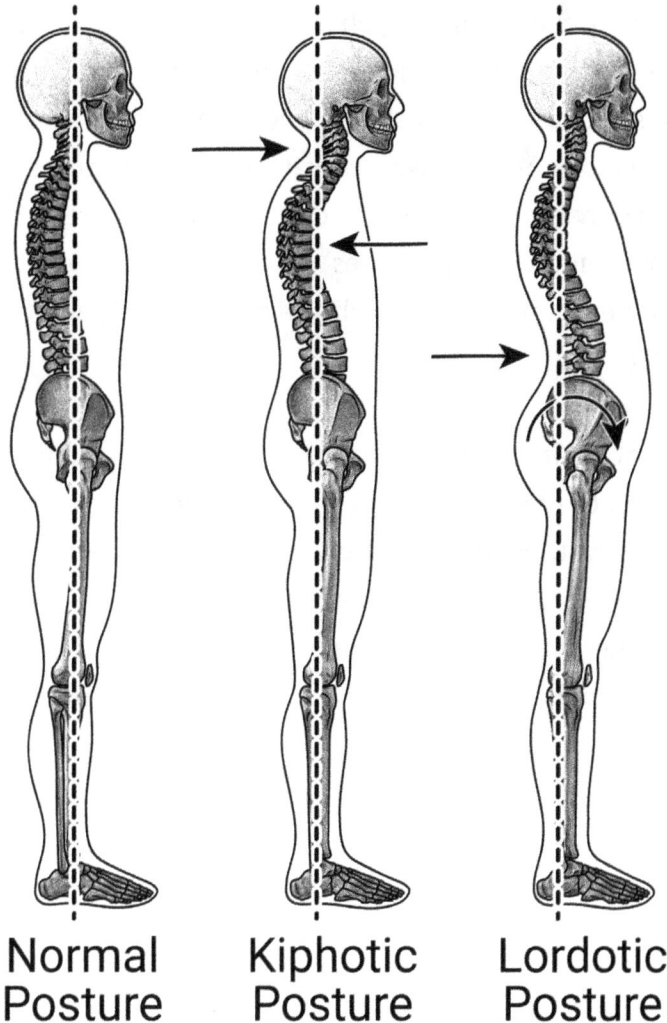

Normal Posture   Kiphotic Posture   Lordotic Posture

Curves with Purpose:

1. **Cervical Spine (Neck):** Your neck should demonstrate a gentle forward curve, placing your head (which weighs close to a bowling ball) in line with your shoulders, your center of gravity. A misalignment here causes a cascade of issues: a forward head posture strains muscles, compresses cervical discs, and has become a silent epidemic in a culture overshadowed by technology screens, as we will explore later.

2. **Thoracic Spine (Upper and Midback):** The thoracic region curves backward in a kyphotic arc, serving as a vital counterbalance to the cervical and lumbar regions. This spring-like structure absorbs shocks and elegantly distributes force as we move. Yet excessive curvature (kyphotic posture), often caused by hunched hours at desks, can lead to structural collapse (compression fractures), compromised respiratory function, and diminished mobility, an unsettling departure from vitality.

3. **Lumbar Spine (Lower Back):** Finally, the lumbar region returns to that forward curve. This lordosis supports the torso's weight, channeling it efficiently down to the pelvis and legs. When this curve is exaggerated, the body's shock absorbers falter, putting intervertebral discs in peril. Lordotic posture heralds potential wear and tear, ticking time bombs for future complications.

Chin tucked, shoulders down and back with a neutral neck

Engaged core with no thoracic extension

Neutral hips and spine posture

The feet should have a strong stable arch. Weight should be distributed evenly

Shoulders rounded with a forward head

Hips forward - anterior pelvic tilt: weak core and glutes

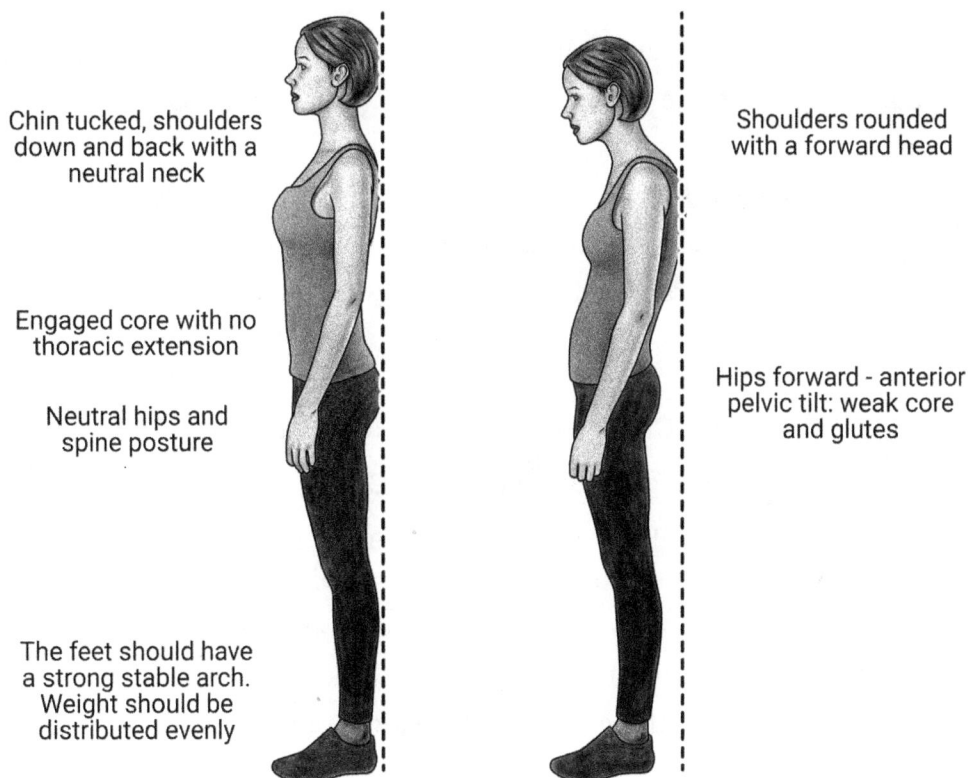

Testing Your Posture Against a Flat Wall

One simple way to evaluate your posture is by using a flat wall as your backdrop. Here's a quick test:

1. Stand with your back against a flat wall, ensuring your heels touch the wall.

2. Bring your shoulder blades together and down, ensuring the middle of your back is in contact with the wall.

3. The back of your head should also be touching the wall. In this position, the ears should align vertically with the shoulders, hips, knees, and ankles, achieving optimal posture.

Check if the natural curves of your spine are maintained. You should be able to fit your hand between the wall and the small of your back without forcing it. If you cannot touch the wall with the back of your head, this could indicate forward head posture.

Taking note of your body's alignment against the wall can provide invaluable feedback on where adjustments might be necessary. Think of it as an ongoing journey, a conscious effort to maintain balance and grace in all we do.

Modern Society: An Architect's Nightmare

We are not living as our geometry intended. Chairs, desks, cars, and smartphones have turned us into slouching, compressed, and often painful versions of ourselves. Sitting for hours on end forces the pelvis into a posterior tilt, flattening the lumbar spine. Staring down at screens transforms our necks into cantilevers, dangling our heads in front of our bodies like wrecking balls. Over time, our tissues adapt to these unnatural positions.

**What begins as a posture problem becomes a structural one—
a remodeling of the body's natural architecture.**

Sitting is the New Smoking

An unfortunate consequence of my desk job is the insidious creep of what is commonly referred to as "sitting disease." And let me tell you, sitting around all day isn't quite as benign as it sounds. Research has shown that prolonged sitting can lead to a series of adverse health effects, much like a silent thief gradually stealing away our vitality. Studies estimate that adults sit for an average of 10 hours a day, a staggering duration that is associated with increased risks of obesity, diabetes, cardiovascular disease, and even early mortality. This result is similar to the ones warned against on cigarette packages!

One of the most glaring issues with sitting for extended periods is its negative impact on posture. Poorly supported bodies slump in their seats, leading to forward head posture, rounded shoulders, and increased strain on the spine. This misalignment doesn't just look unpleasant; it can generate discomfort and exacerbate pre-existing conditions over time.

Sitting, particularly with improper posture, can severely affect the angle of our pelvis and alter the natural lordotic curvature of our spine. When we are seated incorrectly, for instance, with a flattened lower back or slumped shoulders, our pelvis can tilt backward. This shift disrupts the spine's usual curves, leading to an unnatural posture that not only promotes discomfort but can also set the stage for chronic pain and musculoskeletal disorders.

Proper alignment is essential for optimal body mechanics. The lordotic curves of the cervical and lumbar regions, designed to absorb shock and support various movements, falter when the pelvis is misaligned. This misalignment creates a cascade of issues, weakening the muscles that support our upright stance and leading to conditions such as lower back pain, tension, and even degenerative disc disorders.

But that's just the tip of the iceberg. Extended sitting leads to gluteal weakening, a phenomenon that could be dubbed the "dormant butt syndrome." When our powerful glute muscles are left effectively dormant for long periods, they begin to weaken, causing the body to rely more on smaller, stabilizing muscles. This imbalance can trigger myriad problems, including hip discomfort and an increased risk of injury.

The implications of this sitting epidemic extend beyond immediate discomfort; they influence our overall health, longevity, and healthspan. Research shows prolonged sitting is associated with metabolic syndrome, characterized by increased waist circumference, elevated blood pressure, abnormal cholesterol levels, and insulin resistance. These changes subsequently lead to systemic inflammation and serious health conditions. Moreover, studies have indicated that the longer individuals remain sedentary, the greater their likelihood of experiencing cognitive decline.

Addressing the dangers of sitting disease begins with embracing movement. Simple adjustments can dramatically alter our health trajectory. Here are a few practices to integrate into your daily routine:

1. **Take Frequent Breaks:** Aim to stand, stretch, or take a brisk walk every hour. Set reminders on your phone or use an app to keep you accountable. Even a short two-minute walk can break the cycle of stagnation and stimulate circulation.

2. **Desk Ergonomics:** Evaluate your workspace setup. Ensure your chair offers proper lumbar support, and consider using a sit-stand desk to switch positions throughout the day.

3. **Engage Your Glutes:** Implement short exercises that activate your glute muscles during breaks. Simple movements like glute bridges or standing leg lifts can help combat muscle weakness and re-engage your body.

Heads Up: Tackling the Tech Neck Phenomenon

In my daily practice as a neuroradiologist, I frequently encounter a growing trend that seems almost ubiquitous among patients, that is, requests for advanced imaging of neck pain, with CT and MRI scans becoming standard fare. Neck pain, once a fleeting nuisance, has emerged as a common complaint, reflecting the evolution of our lifestyles and the heavy toll that technology takes on our bodies.

As I navigate the demands of my profession, I've not only diagnosed this ailment in others but also experienced its throbbing discomfort and chronic neck tension firsthand. The very nature of my work encourages a forward head posture as I peer at imaging screens for hours on end. While seemingly benign, this subtle shift in posture contributes to a phenomenon increasingly known as "tech neck."

In today's world, many people are glued to their screens, whether working from home, catching up on emails, or enjoying the latest TV series. Prolonged periods of screen time strain the cervical spine, creating persistent tension that affects our necks and overall well-being.

I've witnessed many colleagues walking through the hospital corridors with soft neck braces, newfound badges of honor gifted by orthopedic surgeons, all in a bid to realign their spines and mitigate the pain. The situation is complex; chronic tension can lead to muscle trigger points, those stubborn knots we will discuss that seem to have a life of their own.

Moreover, I've come to recognize that the neck is often the harbor for accumulated stress, the first place to tighten during stressful situations. There's a certain irony in this. As medical professionals, we strive to manage and alleviate the suffering of our patients while battling similar pressures ourselves. This tightening in my neck through stressful weeks reminds me of the intricate connection between physical state and mental strain.

This interplay adds insult to injury, introducing a condition we will discuss: tension myositis syndrome. This syndrome occurs when psychological stress induces chronic muscle changes, particularly in the neck and back, amplifying discomfort and perpetuating a cycle of pain. It's as if our bodies have taken on our emotional burdens, manifesting them physically.

This brings us back to the imaging studies I conduct. The scans often reveal no significant disc herniation, cervical disc degeneration, or arthritic changes in the spine. However, these negative findings can't always capture the postural and emotional narrative behind each patient, how stress, lifestyle choices, and technology dependence converge to create a physical manifestation of pain.

Forward Head Posture:

Let's discuss a major side effect of modern living: the perpetual head bow, as if paying homage to the glowing gods of our screens. Enter the world of Forward Head Posture (FHP), a gift from our digital devotion. Instead of savoring the grace of upright alignment, we unknowingly adopt a forward slump, gently nudged by our tech obsessions.

FHP is more than just an aesthetic concern; it's a gateway to numerous health issues, including neck pain, tension headaches, and the development of bony formations often called "occipital horns" or "text neck." Studies highlight how FHP places undue stress on the cervical spine, resulting in discomfort and potentially leading to degenerative changes over time.

The culprits of Forward Head Posture (FHP) are as common as morning coffee: smartphones enticing us into hours of downward gazes, relentless screen time from watching our favorite streaming services, and perpetual texting routines. These habits coax the head forward, placing undue stress on neck muscles designed to maintain the head's dignified alignment atop the shoulders.

To see a clearer picture, consider this: For every inch your head juts forward, an extra ten pounds of stress is added to your neck and upper back muscles. That's equivalent to hoisting a bowling ball or two! Studies illustrate how modern technology amplifies musculoskeletal strain and leads to cascading health repercussions.

Over time, such forward shifts result in relentless muscle tightness and soreness. If left unchecked, they risk cementing into permanent postural changes, turning tech-induced tendencies into long-term back and neck complaints. Addressing FHP requires awareness and intervention, ensuring a return to the upright posture essential for comfort and health.

This postural pitfall extends beyond adults immersed in technology. Younger individuals, glued to screens from adolescence, also experience shifts in their natural postural alignment. Technology is not inherently detrimental; rather, our unexamined embrace of its conveniences leads to poor posture.

The Conundrum of TMS (Tension Myositis Syndrome):

When considering work-related stress, Tension Myositis Syndrome (TMS) is a condition in which emotional stress manifests as physical pain. It's as if the mind, overwhelmed by life's pressures, transfers its burdens to the body. As a result, areas such as the back, neck, and shoulders can become tight and achy, serving as physical reminders of unexpressed emotions and unresolved stress.

The syndrome is the brain's crafty way of distracting us from emotional turmoil by creating physical discomfort. Think of it as the ultimate avoidance strategy: The problem isn't with your muscles but with an underlying tension that your mind cleverly avoids addressing.

Several studies support the link between stress and physical symptoms, highlighting a crucial connection between our emotional landscape and our bodily experiences. Under stress, the body's fight-or-flight response kicks in, releasing hormones like cortisol and adrenaline to prepare for perceived threats. These same hormones, however, can alter blood flow and increase muscle tension, paving the way for unnecessary pain.

In TMS, blood flow restriction to particular areas leads to muscle and nerve oxygen deprivation, causing discomfort and intense pain. The struggle isn't so much muscular as it is emotional, rooted in stress, anxiety, and repressed feelings. Navigating TMS reminds us of the mind's profound influence on physical well-being.

Muscle Tension to Trigger Points

As we navigate the complex interplay of mind and body tension, we dive deeper into the muscle-tightening world of trigger points. Trigger points are hyperirritable spots within taut bands of skeletal muscle fibers. These tightly contracted areas can cause pain in the immediate region and transfer pain to other parts of the body, a phenomenon known as referred pain. It's not just about unexplained pain, though. Trigger points can limit mobility and functionality. When ignored, they can perpetuate a cycle where tension leads to more stress, trapping muscles in a constant state of contraction.

Scientifically, trigger points form when a muscle experiences sustained contraction or prolonged stress. This leads to local ischemia (a reduction in blood flow due to constriction or blockage) and a subsequent buildup of metabolic byproducts like lactic acid. This ischemia and waste accumulation result in familiar soreness and stiffness, causing further maladaptive signaling within the muscle fibers. This pocket of pain creates a feedback loop in which the muscle continues to contract, perpetuating the problem.

Understanding and addressing trigger points can profoundly improve mobility, comfort, and overall physical well-being. By introducing meticulous movement, targeted release, and a keen awareness of what your body is telling you, you can start to see the human mechanism as a whole again, not as discordant, disparate parts.

Shoulder Pain: Ancient Agility to Modern Constraints

Once upon a time, our ancestors swung gracefully through trees and wielded tools easily, thanks to shoulders built for mobility and strength. Fast forward to today, and many shoulders are, quite literally, in a jam. Changes in our skeleton over millennia, combined with the quirks of modern life, have turned this once-vibrant joint into a common site of pain and dysfunction.

Back in the day, the shoulders of early humans were all about adaptability. Species like Australopithecus or Homo erectus showcased a high, broad scapula and a mobile humeral head. This design was perfect for climbing and reaching, minimizing the risks of shoulder impingement, where our tendons are essentially pinched between our bones. Our ancestors effortlessly climbed trees and used a wide range of motion to support day-to-day survival.

Shoulder Impingement

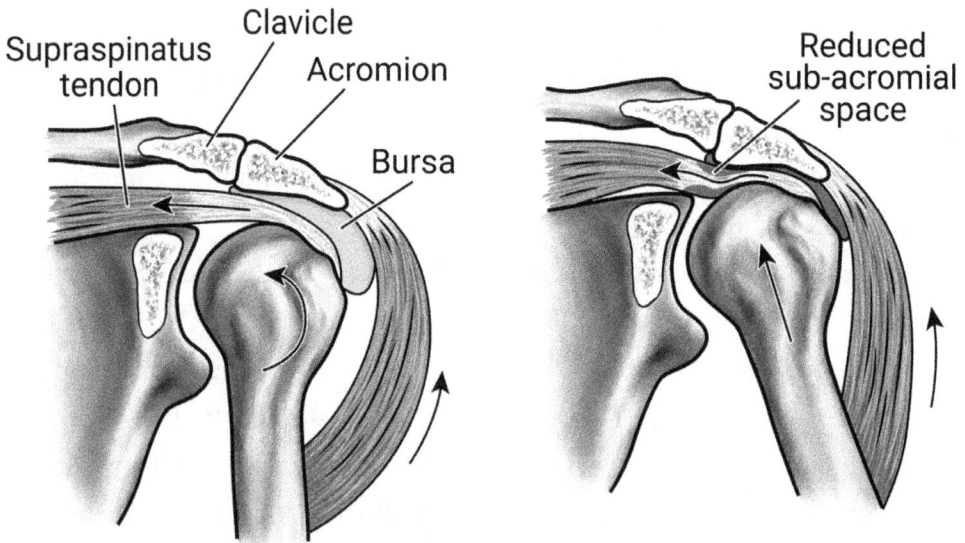

In today's world, many of us are plagued by hunched shoulders and limited movement, thanks to our extended hours spent sitting and leaning forward, whether we're typing at a desk, driving, or scrolling through our smartphones. This change in posture has made our shoulders more vulnerable to injuries. When our shoulders round forward, they effectively squeeze a crucial area called the subacromial space, a small gap beneath the bony prominence at the top of the shoulder. This narrowing can lead to a painful condition known as shoulder impingement, where the tendons in that area get pinched, causing discomfort and restricted movement. Our modern habits tighten this vital space, increasing the likelihood of shoulder pain and injury. Modern postures (forward head tilt, rounded scapulas, and weakened core support) further aggravate the problem. Thanks, technology!

As a radiologist, I see the results of these evolutionary changes. Diagnostic imaging reveals aspects of shoulder evolution and the resulting ailments; X-rays show narrowed spaces between the acromion and humeral head, often with pesky osteophytes (degenerative bone growths) making an appearance. MRI scans reveal thickened tendons, tendinitis, and tears within the rotator cuff. Ultrasound offers real-time visualizations of shoulder movement (or lack thereof), highlighting impingement and dysfunction.

Our shoulders tell a story, from evolutionary triumphs to modern-day trials. Born from a mix of ancient versatility and constrained modernity, they face an uphill battle. However, we can pave a path toward rotator cuff resilience and impingement-free living with knowledge and care.

Crafting Health Through Movement Mastery

In our quest to thrive amidst the technological wonders of modern society, we often find that these very conveniences designed to ease our lives become wrenches jamming our natural gears. Sedentary lifestyles rob us of the essential movements of life—squats, hangs, and carries—that were once the cornerstones of human existence. Without them, we risk a slow atrophy where muscles weaken, bones grow fragile, and the vibrant flow of life is stifled. It's as if our vitality clots, emotions bottle up, and the spark within us fades away.

So, how do we escape this mechanized stagnation and craft a blueprint for optimizing health, longevity, and healthspan? The answer lies in mastering posture and movement from a primal perspective. By connecting with our bodies through movement, we embrace one of the key paradigms for reversing biological age. Movement is not just a remedy for aches; it's a masterful dance with our anatomy, restoring the elegance and strength woven into our very design.

Our bodies are incredible adaptive machines, always striving to adapt to our demands, even if those demands involve countless hours hunched over screens. For a time, we can lean on poor mechanics without visible consequences, but eventually, the reckoning comes. Without proper posture and movement mastery, the body bears the cost of our choices, manifesting in pain and dysfunction. Conversely, by honing our movement, we resolve these issues and enhance our performance and capacity to thrive.

Imagine an athlete in perfect synchronization, every joint and muscle working in concert, a symphony of human mechanics. This mastery is available to all of us when we embrace the foundational principles of biomechanics.

Reflecting on my lineage of master woodworkers, I'm reminded of how form and function were harmonized to craft chairs that support natural spinal alignment. This was about promoting well-being and designing a balance that nurtures comfort and strength. In that same spirit, we aim to restore our innate geometry and natural movement, reclaiming health compromised by life's modern trappings. It's time to celebrate our bodies, revealing the athlete within and embracing the potential of our elegant human architecture.

Functional Movements: Rediscover Your Body's Potential

Welcome to the realm of functional movements, where exercise isn't just about reps and sets but about moving like a human should. Functional movements mimic everyday activities. For example, you might squat to pick up a grocery bag or hang from a tree limb like a kid. These movements use multiple muscle groups, improving strength, balance, flexibility, and coordination in ways that traditional, isolated exercises often miss.

Studies emphasize that exercises that replicate real-life movements can boost functionality and reduce injury risk. By training your body in movements it's designed to perform rather than repetitive, isolated workouts, you create a harmonious balance and improve your practical abilities in everyday life.

Beyond biomechanics, functional exercises are often compound movements that engage multiple joints. Thus, they stimulate the central nervous system more than sitting in a leg extension machine ever could. This multi-joint action improves neuromuscular coordination, benefiting everything from athletic performance to maneuvering through crowded city sidewalks.

Functional movements are not just a physical endeavor; they also cultivate the mind-body connection. When you train using whole-body movements, your brain becomes involved, which improves mental acuity and focus. Each compound movement enhances proprioception, the awareness of your body in space. This alignment of mind and movement is crucial for avoiding the injuries commonly associated with traditional workouts. You're less likely to push past your limits when you're in tune with your body's movements.

Ultimately, functional movements are about building a more durable, agile version of yourself, armed with the strength, flexibility, and coordination to handle life's challenges gracefully and efficiently. They're your ticket to maintaining independence longer, ensuring you can reach for that can on the top shelf, lift a grandchild, or simply enjoy the freedom of movement. Functional movement is less about exercise and more about life and enhancing your human experience to be strong, capable, and resilient.

By aligning our bodies with primal patterns, we can address the pitfalls of a sedentary lifestyle and reclaim health, vitality, and timeless resilience. Let's explore these essential movements, understanding their significance and applications in our quest to reverse biological age.

1. Squatting

Relevance: Squatting is one of the most fundamental human actions. For everyone from toddlers to Olympians, squats engage your quads, glutes, and calves while activating your core for support. Squatting is more than just a gym rep; it's a foundational human movement essential for activities like sitting, standing, and lifting. Imagine our ancestors squatting to forage or rest.

Benefits: Squats bolster leg strength, enhance hip mobility, and fortify core stability while promoting joint health.

Applications: Delve into deep squats to enhance mobility, air squats for bodyweight training, or add resistance to increase challenge and strength.

2. Hinging
Relevance: This movement mimics the bending motions needed to lift objects, such as gathering firewood or hoisting a child.

Benefits: Hinging is crucial for strengthening the posterior chain (glutes, hamstrings, and lower back) and is key to preventing back injuries.

Applications: Engage in deadlifts, kettlebell swings, and good mornings to master hinging mechanics and build robust support.

3. Hanging
Relevance: Rooted in primal tasks like climbing and carrying, these movements reflect our ancestors' dynamic activities. Essentially, it is an upper-body stretch and strength fest.

Benefits: Strengthens your shoulders, core, forearms, and grip while decompressing your spine, a trifecta that helps counteract modern life's lousy posture and imbalances.

Applications: Consider hanging for a few minutes daily as a reset button for your upper body.

4. Sprinting
Relevance: Imagine our ancestors on the hunt, charging at prey

with all their might and then cooling down in anticipation of the next opportunity.

Benefits: These activities bolster cardiovascular health, enhance balance and coordination, and build endurance.

Applications: Incorporate sprint intervals for intensity in your cardio workout.

5. Rotational Movements
Relevance: Twisting for tasks is an intrinsic movement vital for throwing and reaching activities.

Benefits: These movements boost core strength, spinal mobility, and athletic prowess.

Applications: Practice Russian twists, woodchoppers, and medicine ball throws to encourage dynamic core engagement.

6. Carrying
Relevance: These practical exercises mimic the ancestral tasks of carrying water and supplies.

Benefits: Carrying develops full-body strength, grip endurance, and resilience. Weighted carries can build core stability and improve posture by activating large muscle groups essential for coordination and balance.

Applications: To build strength and endurance, explore farmer's and suitcase carries or challenge yourself with sandbag carries.

7. Jumping and Landing

Relevance: Essential for survival tactics like climbing or escaping, these movements demand precision and power.

Benefits: Jump-related activities build explosive power, improve coordination, and strengthen bones, essential for active living.

Applications: Master box jumps, broad jumps, or other plyometric drills for dynamic movement.

8. Balancing

Relevance: When navigating natural terrain or urban landscapes, balance is crucial.

Benefits: Enhances stability, proprioception, and core muscular endurance.

Applications: Challenge yourself with single-leg balance drills, yoga, or balancing on natural elements.

9. Stretching and Mobility

Relevance: Reflects natural motions like reaching or climbing, which are essential for functional movement.

Benefits: Improves flexibility, boosts joint health, and supports better posture.

Applications: Enhance mobility by engaging in dynamic stretches, yoga poses, or primal flows like Animal Flow (ground-based quadrupedal movement program).

10. Breath Work

Relevance: Breath control is paramount at the core of survival and peak performance.

Benefits: Manage stress, optimize energy, and support respiratory health.

Applications: Practice diaphragmatic breathing or box breathing. More on this in Chapter 4.

As we integrate these primal movements into our routines, let us do so mindfully. Feel your body reconnecting with its innate design, awakening strength, and embracing resilience. This reconnection with our evolutionary origins invites physical rejuvenation and a deeper understanding of bodily fluency, a key to reversing biological age.

Rucking: The Backpack Adventure

Having just traversed the world of functional movements where every squat and hang reconnects us to our primal roots, it's time to gear up for a journey that takes natural movement to the next level. Welcome to the world of rucking.

Rucking, at its heart, is elegantly simple: the act of walking with a weighted backpack or vest. Sounds too easy, right? Well, this isn't just a stroll in the park; it's a full-body workout born from necessity and steeped in history. Remember those childhood days when carrying your school backpack seemed akin to a military operation? Turns out, you were onto something.

The practice has many benefits. It is modeled after our ancestors' need to routinely carry heavy loads over varied terrains. Rucking harks back to times when life involved carrying essentials, whether the day's kill, firewood, or children. It combines cardio, strength, and resilience training, offering an adaptable workout that enhances endurance and muscle tone without the intensity (or intimidation) of running.

Contemporary research highlights how rucking can burn significant calories while improving cardiovascular health. Studies show that rucking with moderate weight increases caloric burn by up to 30% compared to regular walking. Moreover, it engages core muscles, fortifying back and shoulder strength, while the added weight naturally improves bone density, a key factor for long-term health.

Rucking is a nod to an era when every village errand or hunting trip involved carrying some load. It rekindles the muscle memory and resilience built over millennia, encouraging a movement that aligns the body with function. By shouldering your pack, you join the ranks of those travelers who moved with purpose, bonding with the Earth's rhythms and utilizing what nature offered.

Rucking requires no special gym membership or expensive equipment. All that's needed is a backpack and some creativity; start light, using books or water bottles, and gradually increase the weight as your stamina builds. Begin with shorter distances, focusing on maintaining good posture and ensuring the backpack is snug and supported close to your body. Rucking invites you to rediscover the simplicity and depth of putting one foot in front of the other, weighted with intent.

Rucking to Running: Reversing Cardiovascular Age

As we lighten our loads from the world of rucking, it's time to pick up the pace and embrace a practice that taps into our ancient instinct to sprint and recover. Imagine our ancestors on the hunt, charging after prey with all their might, then cooling down as they awaited the next opportunity. This cycle of intense effort followed by rest was nature's original form of High-Intensity Interval Training (HIIT). It sent strong epigenetic signals to their cardiovascular systems, promoting sharpness and resilience.

These bursts of intense activity, followed by periods of rest, fashioned a powerful framework for heart health. Such was the dance between rest and rigor that it prepped our cardiovascular systems for the peaks and valleys of prehistoric life. Fast forward to today, and this age-old exercise pattern is expertly captured in the Norwegian Protocol, a modern approach tapping into HIIT to rejuvenate heart health.

The Science of the Norwegian Protocol

The Norwegian Protocol is a specific HIIT regimen designed to mimic these bursts and recoveries, consisting of four-minute intervals at 85% to 95% of your maximum heart rate, alternated with three-minute active recovery periods. This protocol boosts fitness and reverses cardiovascular age. Imagine wiping years off your heart by embracing tactics that awaken your core!

The protocol's intrigue lies in its ability to promote changes at a cellular level. Optimally stretching cardiac muscles and enhancing blood flow rejuvenates the endothelial cells, those critical gatekeepers of vascular health, leading to improved oxygen uptake and circulation while lowering blood pressure and resting heart rates.

By diving into HIIT, we channel our ancestors' primal interactions, reigniting a physiological conversation with our genes meant to fortify the body's network for survival. As our forebears pursued their quarry, their bodies instinctively adjusted—harder and faster on sprints, then slower to rest, during which cardiovascular improvements took root.

During HIIT sessions today, from stationary bikes to treadmills, we practically walk in their footsteps. It's about not only achieving peaks of power but also allowing time for the body's systems to recalibrate in those recovery moments. The magic happens in the surge and soothing respite, a holistic balance that returns to primal rhythms.

For modern adopters, think variety; mix up your hiking trail sprints with interval cycling or rowing. Monitor heart rates using fitness trackers, and pay attention to the balance between exertion and rest, ensuring it promotes physical harmony, much like a well-conducted orchestra.

The beauty of the Norwegian HIIT method lies in harmony, the marrying of ancient heart wisdom with modern science's finesse. It amplifies cardiovascular capacity, reminding us that health transpires not through relentless, steady motion but through embracing fluctuations, celebrating both dynamism and recovery.

Joint Longevity and Mobility

Our joints are the connectors that allow us to navigate the world; without them, even the simplest movements would be impossible. It's essential to prioritize mobility and joint integrity to maintain physical function and actively reverse biological age. As we age, joints can become stiff and susceptible to wear and tear, leading to discomfort and reduced mobility. However, ample research indicates that regular mobility drills, active stretching, and strengthening exercises can help mitigate these effects. By prioritizing joint health, we enable our bodies to move fluidly and maintain youthful vitality.

Controlled Articular Rotations (CARs):

One effective method of enhancing joint mobility is controlled articular rotations (CARs). These slow, controlled movements target a joint's full range of motion, promoting synovial fluid circulation and joint health. This technique allows for greater awareness of movement mechanics and helps identify any restrictions or tightness in the joint. Regular practice of CARs aids in maintaining and restoring joint function, fostering resilience that stands the test of time.

Dynamic Flexibility Exercises:

Dynamic flexibility exercises are another powerful tool in promoting joint longevity. Unlike static stretches, dynamic movements incorporate controlled exercises that take joints through their full range of motion while simulating everyday activities. These exercises engage multiple muscle groups while preparing the body for more dynamic movement patterns, ultimately enhancing joint function and stability.

Animal Yoga:

Have you ever heard of animal yoga? It's an engaging practice that incorporates movements mimicking those of various animals. Think downward dog or pigeon pose. This approach adds playfulness to your routine and pulls from our primal behaviors, tapping into the functional movements that kept our ancestors agile and strong. Using techniques inspired by animal movements, practitioners can reestablish natural mobility and flexibility, reconnecting with the raw mechanics of human movement. This protects and restores joints and harmonizes the body's active dynamic with the fluidity of animal-inspired flow.

Research backs the assertion that engaging in regular mobility and flexibility exercises can positively affect bone and joint health. When we move through life with agility and grace, our biological systems respond positively, weaving together the fabric of holistic health. Joint longevity isn't just a matter of keeping our bodies functional; it's a proactive strategy to enrich our lives and extend our years of vitality.

The Body-Breath Connection

In my late 20s, I underwent the classic rite of passage: wisdom teeth removal. Several months later, I began to notice, or rather, people around me noticed, a change. My breathing had gotten louder, and friends and family tactfully suggested I might have nasal issues. Fast-forward to my 40s and I found myself battling bouts of extreme fatigue and drowsiness. My doctor pointed out that my crowded teeth needed to be addressed, recommending braces.

Now, picture this: I'm a radiologist, spending my day dictating reports. Traditional braces felt like a medieval device that affected my speech, so I exchanged them for clear aligners. That's when things got even trickier. My breathing took a nosedive, with nighttime episodes of choking and sweat-drenched awakenings. Enter Dr. M, my astute restorative dentist. We unearthed the root of it all with her insight: a small arch, a casualty of the evolution of modern man.

Modern human mouths have changed dramatically compared to those of our ancestors, and it's not all for the better. In ancient times, our human forebears had strong jaws and a full set of healthy teeth perfectly designed for their primal diet of tough, fibrous vegetation and raw meats. Their diets required robust chewing, strengthening the jaw, shaping the dental arch, and positioning the teeth optimally for both function and form. The act of chewing these fibrous foods promoted proper jaw development, resulting in wider arches and better airway space.

Fast forward to today, and our dietary habits have shifted dramatically. The introduction of processed foods (think soft breads, sugary snacks, and other easily consumable items) has dramatically softened our diets. This lack of necessary chewing has repercussions that extend beyond mere dental aesthetics. The resultant narrowing of the dental arch contributes to breathing issues, creating a landscape predisposed to sleep apnea and other respiratory complications.

Dr. M explained that extracting my wisdom teeth while having a naturally narrow arch compromised my throat space, exacerbating my breathing woes and ushering in borderline sleep apnea. Her solution? A custom series of aligners to widen my mouth arch and restore balance. It worked wonders. My breathing improved dramatically, my sleep was no longer a midnight wrestling match, and I could say goodbye to my daytime lethargy.

This personal saga reminds us of how modern lifestyles have inadvertently reshaped something as essential as our breathing. While a person's dental structure may seem like a minor detail in the grand scheme of health, it serves as a critical reminder that even the evolution of our mouths and teeth is intrinsically linked to holistic health. The interplay of diet, dental architecture, and airway integrity reveals a larger narrative about reclaiming our well-being by addressing our primal needs, wisdom often overshadowed in a world fixated on convenience.

A Neuroradiologist's Perspective on Skull Evolution

Picture cracking open a time capsule to reveal the profound ways in which human skulls have evolved. From the robust cranial structures of ancient humans to the more delicate forms we see today, this evolution has significantly impacted our health, especially our ability to breathe. The skull is like a map for a radiologist, charting the journey from ancient adaptability to modern-day complexities.

Radiology offers insights into how our modern diet and lifestyle have reshaped our skull anatomy and our well-being.

Skull Shape and Size:

Take a peek inside the skull of an ancient human, say Homo erectus, and you'll notice a fortress-like cranial structure. With larger jaws, prominent brow ridges, and thicker bones, these folks were equipped for the rigors of a hunter-gatherer lifestyle, with the tools to tackle tough, fibrous foods.

Fast forward to today, and you'll find our skulls have slimmed down as if they've been on a diet too. Our lighter, fragile skulls feature shorter faces and smaller jaws, a testament to modern conveniences and softer diets that lack the intense mastication required in the past. Smaller nasal passages and a down-sized maxilla aren't just signposts of evolution; they're culprits in the rising tide of respiratory issues like sleep apnea.

Jaw and Dental Arch Reduction:

Our ancestors possessed jaws with the confidence of a linebacker, bulky and rugged, perfect for chomping raw, untamed vittles. This constant chewing gave jaw muscles a workout and maintained wide dental arches, keeping the airway clear and the breath unencumbered.

Contrast that with today's smaller, narrower jaws, contorted by a life of processed food and softer bites, and you'll see why teeth crowd into that dreaded lineup of misalignment. The crowding reduces tongue space, and when combined with a narrower airway, it's a perfect storm for obstructive sleep apnea.

Breathing Patterns

Our ancestors were likely masters of nasal breathing, benefitting from larger nasal passages that provided humidification, filtration, and improved oxygen exchange. The modern shift to mouth breathing, due in part to smaller sinuses and jaw structures, can increase airway blockage risk, degrade air quality, and possibly exacerbate sleep apnea.

Sedentary Lifestyles and Posture

Add our modern sedentary lifestyle (a stark contrast to the active life of ancient humans, with strong posture and efficient respiratory function) to the mix and you get weaker respiratory muscles and out-of-sync airways, especially when coupled with the prevalence of "tech neck."

Radiological imaging serves as a window into these structural shifts. Lateral skull radiographs often highlight smaller jaws and sunken facial bones, contributing to a narrower airway and more frequent episodes of obstructive sleep apnea. CT scans often reveal smaller nasal and sinus cavities in contemporary skulls versus their ancient counterparts, along with airways that occasionally collapsed as the patients lay supine on the scanner table. Understanding and addressing the anatomical intricacies revealed through imaging can help us better navigate these health challenges. Modern living may have reshaped our skulls, but with attention and action, we can redesign how we breathe and thrive.

Rethinking Our Approach

Myofunctional Therapy: Involves exercises that strengthen facial and tongue muscles, support the airways, and promote nasal breathing. These exercises may help alleviate sleep apnea.

Restorative Orthodontics: Involves treatments that expand dental arches, creating more space for the tongue and encouraging proper airflow.

Mewing Exercises: Mewing is a technique that focuses on the way you position your tongue in your mouth. It comes from Dr. John Mew, the orthodontist who developed the method. The idea is simple: you place your tongue flat against the roof of your mouth. This practice helps shape and support your facial structure, improve your breathing, and create more space in your airway. By consistently maintaining this proper tongue posture, you can encourage healthier jawline development and promote better oral health. Think of it as a natural way to train your mouth and improve how you look and breathe!

Reviving Body Wisdom: From Ancient Awareness to Modern Reconnections

In the days of ancient humans, life was a high-stakes game of awareness, the kind that kept you sharp but agile as you dodged predators or foraged for sustenance. Back then, staying in tune with your body was a survival instinct honed to perfection. Fast-forward to today, and this primal connection has frayed, overtaken by our cozy, tech-laden worlds. But fear not! Modern man can restore this essential relationship by blending ancient practices and contemporary science.

Tai Chi: The Dance of Balance

Enter Tai Chi, an ancient martial art that isn't just about graceful moves but is a ticket to balance, flexibility, and mental clarity. Think of it as meditation in motion, where each slow, deliberate movement fosters a deep connection to the body. Studies indicate that Tai Chi enhances balance and flexibility and significantly reduces stress and the risk of falls.

Studies have shown that the practice of Tai Chi reduces falls in older adults compared to those who do not practice. By engaging in the rhythmic movements of Tai Chi, practitioners tune into their body's cues, promoting a harmonious body-mind connection that staves off some of the physical pitfalls of aging.

Proprioception: The Inner Compass

Proprioception is the body's internal GPS, a remarkable sense that tells us where we are in space. Improving proprioception can lead to fewer injuries and more precise movements, marked perks for anyone looking to up their game or simply navigate daily life more safely. Athletes and dancers often excel in this sensory art, but you don't have to star in a Broadway show to benefit.

Exercise regimes, including balance training and yoga, can boost proprioceptive acuity by focusing on aligning muscle and joint function with neural signals. This bolstered body awareness helps individuals maneuver with enhanced control, improving functionality and reducing injury risk.

Interoception: The Language of the Body

Interoception is more subtle than balance and spatial awareness. It is the perception of physiological signals within the body, akin to learning a language that's been whispering inside us all along. From hunger pangs to the gentle internal hum you feel during meditation, interoception informs how we interpret and respond to our body's needs.

A well-attuned interoceptive system can improve emotional regulation and improve health outcomes. Studies have linked strong interoceptive awareness to better stress management and fewer anxiety disorders, as individuals become more adept at interpreting bodily signals well before they escalate into discomfort.

Rebuilding the Bridge

So, how do we embark on this journey to rekindle the refined bodily awareness of ancient times? We embrace practices like Tai Chi for flow, seek exercises that enhance proprioception for internal cues, and listen closely to interoceptive signals for profound insights into our well-being.

By reviving these ancient connections and marrying them with modern insights, we can tune back into our bodies' rhythms. This not only leads to enhanced health and reduced injury risks but also encourages a life led with intuition and balance, rekindling the wisdom of those who walked this earth eons before us.

Embracing our Body's Primal Intelligence

As we conclude this chapter, we are reminded of the intricate wisdom our bodies hold. The Hadzabe engaged in daily activities such as hunting and gathering and maintained functional movement patterns that enhanced their health, balance, and flexibility. Their movements often involved overhead activities, such as throwing spears or carrying heavy loads, that naturally promoted shoulder strength and reduced pain, a stark contrast to modern society's sedentary, rounded posture.

We discussed the benefits of practices like rucking, a modern adaptation that mirrors primal activities like carrying a kill or other heavy loads. Walking with weights improves bone density, joint stability, and muscular endurance, contributing to longevity and reverse biological aging. Likewise, the high-intensity bursts of effort required in hunts parallel the benefits of modern HIIT protocols, like the Norwegian 4x4, which mimic this primal pattern of exertion and rest, optimizing cardiovascular health and metabolic efficiency.

The primal man demonstrated predominant nasal breathing, a habit formed by sufficient jaw and airway development due to their diets rich in unprocessed, fibrous foods. Modern soft diets have led to underdeveloped jaws and issues like mouth breathing and sleep apnea. However, restorative practices such as myofunctional therapy, chewing exercises, and orthodontic interventions can help counteract these effects, restoring efficient breathing patterns and enhancing oxygen delivery to the body.

Additionally, modern life's reliance on technology has introduced challenges like forward head posture and "tech neck," leading to spinal misalignment and muscular imbalances. Counteracting these requires active engagement in postural correction, strengthening neck muscles, and maintaining alignment. Our environment's chronic stressors also contribute to conditions like tension myositis syndrome and muscle trigger points. Techniques like myofascial release, mindfulness, and breathwork are essential for addressing these.

To deepen our connection with the body, practices like Tai Chi, proprioception training, and interoception exercises, which heighten internal body awareness, can be transformative. These methods foster harmony between mind and body, helping us attune to subtle cues from within and promote self-healing.

While modern life imposes unique challenges on our skeletal, muscular, and respiratory systems, we can reclaim our health. By embracing primal health practices, we align ourselves with our evolutionary design, empowering us to navigate the demands of contemporary living with resilience and vitality.

You're not a slave to modernity. You can rebuild your human architecture, one habit, one stretch, one moment of awareness at a time. The blueprint is already inside you. All you have to do is remember how to use it.

Primal Practices:

1. Mindful Movement & Functional Exercises:

Incorporate exercises into your routine that enhance core strength and promote balanced movement. Daily tasks can become opportunities for movement; for instance, practice squatting while picking up items around the house. Find a sturdy bar or branch and hang for a minute to help decompress your spine and build shoulder strength.

2. Weekly Rucking:

Make rucking a regular part of your week; strap on a backpack with some weight and take a brisk walk outdoors. Not only does this strengthen your body, but it also improves bone density.

3. Posture Check:

Be mindful of your posture throughout the day. Stand tall, imagining a string gently pulling you upward from the crown of your head. This encourages even weight distribution and combats the effects of forward head posture, often tied to tech use.

4. Digital Detox:

Schedule regular breaks from screens to reconnect with the world around you. Use this time to engage in activities that naturally lift your gaze; take a walk, chat with a friend, or simply breathe in nature's beauty. This practice helps maintain a neutral neck position, reducing strain and tension.

5. Ergonomic Allies:

Evaluating your workspace is crucial in combating tech-induced posture issues. To encourage healthier screen interactions, elevate your monitors to eye level and utilize ergonomic tools like laptop stands and external keyboards. Additionally, elevating your smartphone can help prevent the chronic downward gaze. By acknowledging the modern pull toward poor posture and actively working to strengthen and realign, we can stave off the negative consequences of forward head posture (FHP).

6. Neck Strengthening Exercises: Reclaim Your Natural Posture

Focus on reinforcing your neck muscles. Neck exercises counterbalance forward head posture. Isometric exercises (pressing your head softly against your palm in various directions, for example) help strengthen neck muscles. Pair these with gentle neck stretches and the "chin tuck," which involves moving your chin inward to elongate the neck and realign the spine. These practices promote stability, resilience, and support for your neck.

7. Mindfulness and Meditation:

Include mindfulness practices in your daily routine to ground yourself in the present moment. Mental space is crucial for reducing stress; consider integrating meditation sessions that allow your mind to declutter and your body to relax.

8. Myofascial Release

A manual therapy technique for relaxing contracted muscles, improving blood flow, and stimulating the muscle stretch reflex, this technique uses sustained pressure and stretching to loosen tension and iron out those unsightly wrinkles in your body's soundscape.

Massage therapists and trained practitioners work to identify trigger points and use their fingers, knuckles, or elbows to apply pressure, unwinding the knotted bands and smoothing out the discord.

9. Physical Awareness Practices:

Enhance body awareness through Tai Chi or similar gentle movement practices. These methods encourage mindfulness and help to release tension that accumulates in the muscles.

10. Foam Rolling and Stretching:

Implement foam rolling in your self-care routine. It's an effective tool for self-myofascial release, applying pressure to trigger points and relieving muscle tightness. Pair this with regular stretching exercises to maintain flexibility and ensure the muscles stay pliable.

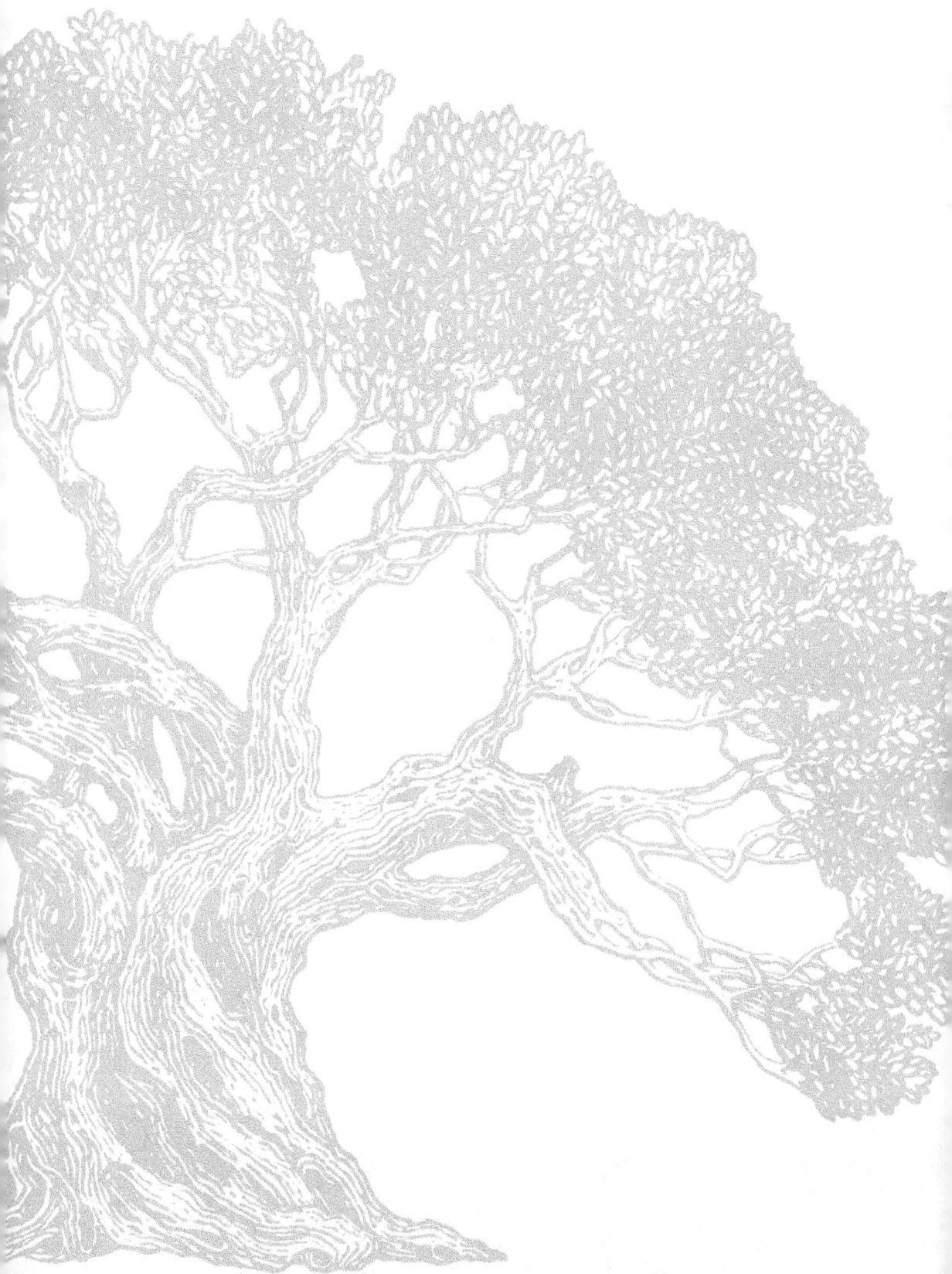

3

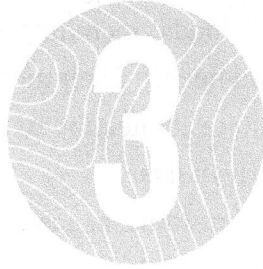

NOURISHING BONDS:
CULTIVATING A CONNECTION WITH FOOD

*"When we nourish our bodies with intention, we nourish
our connection to the earth, our ancestors, and the life
force that sustains us."*
– Kavin Misty, MD

Imagine little me, running barefoot alongside the Hadzabe children, reveling in the joy of unstructured play in the great outdoors. While I was busy playing, the other kids casually scoured the earth for grasshoppers to catch. They would fill tin cans with these critters and toss in some dried leaves, setting the stage for what I could only describe as a bug-treat party. They'd burn the leaves and roast the bugs while I stood back, determined to resist the challenge. Despite their playful prodding, I could never bring myself to eat a whole grasshopper; my teenage taste buds weren't quite ready for that leap into entomophagy! I pretended to take a bite and discreetly discarded the evidence.

Looking back, I realize those experiences were filled with valuable lessons about food and health. Today, there's a growing acknowledgment of how traditional and primal diets contribute to lower incidences of chronic diseases in these tribes. Research highlights that the Hadzabes' dietary patterns, heavily reliant on nutrient-dense local foods, including tubers rich in prebiotic fiber, significantly bolster their overall health. Their mealtimes were spontaneous and unregimented. They had an innate connection to food that many of us have lost in our modern, convenience-driven lives.

The Hadzabe also practice intermittent fasting, driven by food availability rather than rigid dietary schedules. This approach, coupled with their active lifestyle, supports metabolic health and illustrates a functional and intuitive way of eating. Their diet, devoid of processed foods, is a natural remedy for inflammation and disease, echoing the knowledge verified by current health research.

As we embark on this chapter, let us explore how we can cultivate a rich connection with food that reflects the wisdom of the Hadzabe and other primal communities. By integrating nutrient-dense foods, practicing mindful eating, and reconnecting with the earth's bounty, we can nourish our bodies to optimize our health and honor our roots.

Join me as we delve into the transformational power of food and its ability to strengthen our nourishing bonds with ourselves, our communities, and the natural world around us. Let's rediscover how food can provide vitality, joy, and deep connection in our journey to optimal health.

The Hadzabe: Guardians of Ancient Wisdom

At the heart of Hadzabe culture is a profound understanding of and respect for nature. They spend their days hunting small game with bows and arrows and foraging for edible plants, tubers, and fruits. The seasons dictate their diet, which aligns naturally with what the environment provides. This lifestyle is environmentally sustainable and ideally in sync with nature's cycles.

The Hadzabe men typically hunt, often supplementing their diet with honey from wild beehives, while the women gather tubers and berries. This communal effort ensures nutritional diversity drawn directly from their ancestral knowledge. Perhaps these seasonal cycles and diverse diets contribute to the Hadzabes' remarkable health and vitality, with records showing a low incidence of diabetes, heart disease, and other chronic conditions that plague industrialized societies.

In recent years, the Hadzabe have caught the eye of longevity researchers curious to understand their secrets of health and endurance. Scientists studying the tribe have highlighted their impressive cardiovascular health and metabolic flexibility, remarkable for a society without access to modern healthcare. Their active lifestyle and high-fiber diet are believed to contribute to their strong hearts and robust health.

The Hadzabes' hunter-gatherer way of life has become a point of interest for those studying how lifestyle influences longevity. Their flexibility in diet, rich in fiber and low in processed foods, supports a healthy gut microbiome, which is critical for reducing inflammation and promoting overall health. This connection between lifestyle and health provides a compelling argument against our fast-food, high-stress lifestyles.

For anyone seeking lessons in living well, the Hadzabe offer a masterclass in simplicity and sustainability. Their ability to harness the land's provisions seasonally, eat mindfully, and remain active outdoors reminds us of the power of returning to basics.

As modern reporting highlights tribes like the Hadzabe, it emphasizes that perhaps we can invite a little of their ethos into our lives, appreciating the mutual relationship we can have with nature, ensuring balance and health are woven into the fabric of daily existence. The Hadzabe quietly remind us that while the world evolves, some wisdom remains timeless.

Intermittent Fasting: Aligning with Ancestral Rhythms

Reflecting on my time with the Hadzabe tribe, one of the most fascinating aspects of their lifestyle was their natural approach to eating, sometimes seemingly dictated by the whims of nature rather than rigid schedules. While they celebrated their foraging successes with a feast, there were also moments of scarcity that led them to fast. This effortless ebb and flow of feasting and fasting is worth exploring, especially as we delve into the science behind intermittent fasting and its myriad health benefits.

Intermittent fasting (IF) and time-restricted eating mimic the Hadzabes' natural rhythms. In the wild, our ancestors didn't have the luxury of three square meals daily. Instead, they adapted to the availability of food, which meant periods of plenty followed by times of scarcity. This evolutionary basis for fasting has equipped humans with a survival strategy that allows the body to switch gears based on external conditions.

Research demonstrates that fasting triggers autophagy, a cellular cleanup process that removes damaged cells and regenerates healthy ones. This biological reboot is akin to hitting the refresh button on your computer, ensuring all systems run more smoothly and efficiently. As we apply this ancient wisdom in modern contexts, it becomes clear that intermittent fasting isn't just a trend, it's a powerful tool for enhancing metabolic health.

Scientific studies reveal that intermittent fasting can significantly improve insulin sensitivity, one of the key players in metabolic function. Enhanced insulin sensitivity allows cells to absorb glucose more effectively, resulting in lower blood sugar levels and a reduced risk of type 2 diabetes. This cycle of fasting and feasting also lowers inflammation, which has become a standard bearer for numerous chronic ailments in our society.

Furthermore, research indicates that the benefits extend to brain health. Intermittent fasting has been linked to neuroprotection, shielding our neurons from age-related decline and promoting cognitive resilience. **Taking a little time away from food helps your brain improve, demonstrating that our bodies thrive on balance and cycles.**

The Hadzabe tribe's intuitive approach to eating reminds us that embracing our evolutionary heritage can guide us toward better health. While ultra-processed foods and constant snacking have become staples in modern diets, we can learn from these primal cultures. We can foster a more harmonious relationship with food and, ultimately, our overall health by weaving intermittent fasting into our routines, whether through time-restricted eating or simply allowing longer breaks between meals.

So, as you ponder your meals, remember that sometimes less is more. Each fasting moment can be a step toward rejuvenation and vitality, a connection to our past that empowers our future. Embrace this timeless practice, and you might find your body thanking you in ways you never thought possible.

The Science of the Gut Microbiome: The Hidden Powerhouse Within

Imagine your gut as an elaborate metropolis with trillions of residents, microbes like bacteria, viruses, fungi, and other tiny dwellers, all thriving in your digestive tract. This vibrant community, often called the "second brain," is crucial for maintaining overall health and impacts everything from digestion to immunity and mood.

Your gut microbiome is like a unique fingerprint shaped by genetics, diet, and lifestyle. Research reveals that greater microbial diversity correlates with better health outcomes. People enriched with varied gut bacteria show lower levels of inflammation and a reduced risk of chronic diseases such as diabetes and obesity.

Feeding your gut a fiber-rich diet is like rolling out a red carpet for these beneficial bacteria. Prebiotics, such as inulin in foods like onions and garlic, serve as dietary fuel for these microbes, enhancing their activity and diversity. As these microbes thrive, they produce short-chain fatty acids (SCFAs), which are vital in regulating the immune system and reducing inflammation.

An astounding 70% of our immune cells reside in the gut, highlighting it as a pivotal player in immune response. A balanced microbiome modulates immune functions, effectively guiding the body in distinguishing between allies and invaders. The gut microbiome's communication with the immune system helps fine-tune responses, fostering resilient immunity.

Prepare yourself for a fascinating twist: Your gut and brain are constantly conversing. This is facilitated through pathways like the vagus nerve and neurotransmitter production. Some gut bacteria generate serotonin, a key neurotransmitter influencing mood and emotional balance. This bidirectional communication implies that a healthy gut can significantly impact mental health, potentially boosting mood and cognitive function.

To leverage the powerhouse within, focus on fostering microbial diversity through a diet rich in prebiotics and probiotics. Consider this approach a dietary adjustment and a comprehensive strategy to enhance overall health, revealing the microbiome's extensive role in the body's ecosystem.

Gut Microbiome and Primal Diets

In Africa, I noticed that hunter-gatherers like the Hadzabe lived intimately connected to their environment, and their diet was a vibrant reflection of the land around them. Constantly exposed to a rich tapestry of nature, they consumed a variety of foods. Still, the tubers, particularly yucca, stood out as a source of prebiotic fiber essential in fostering a robust gut microbiome.

When studying the gut microbiome, the contrasting dietary habits between modern humans and hunter-gatherers provide valuable insights. Hunter-gatherers like the Hadzabe consume fiber-rich diets, ultimately supporting a more diverse gut microbiome. Scientific research indicates that this diversity is a bellwether for health, equipping our microbiomes with the power to reduce inflammation, improve digestion, and bolster immune function.

So, what makes these varied foods so crucial? Prebiotic fibers, like those found in tubers and fibrous fruits, provide food for beneficial gut bacteria, feeding the vibrant community necessary for a healthy system. When our modern diets rely on fast, processed foods that lack sufficient fiber, we inadvertently starve our beneficial bacteria, leading to a less diverse microbiome. A well-fed microbiome is like a thriving city; the more diverse the inhabitants, the more resilient the community, ready to fend off threats and keep the peace.

Conversely, the Hadzabes' traditional diet ensures access to prebiotic-rich foods and naturally fermented items that nurture their gut flora. Fermented foods containing probiotics, those delightful, living microbes, help maintain gut health by adding beneficial bacteria directly into the mix. Think of these foods as a security team, fortifying the city's defenses against invaders.

A varied microbiome enhances the gut's ability to digest different substances efficiently, further supporting overall nutrient assimilation. Healthy gut ecosystems lead to improved digestion and nutrient absorption, key elements for vitality and wellness.

In contrast, the modern diet, laden with processed foods and lacking a diversity of prebiotic fibers, has been linked to a host of health issues, including obesity, diabetes, and gastrointestinal disorders. The stark differences between the Hadzabe and modern eating patterns illustrate the consequences of dietary choices on our resilient little companions within.

With a mindful approach to diet, taking cues from ancient practices, we can cultivate vibrant gut health, unlocking physical resilience and well-being. Just as my experiences with the Hadzabe tribe taught me the importance of living in harmony with our food, so too can we infuse our modern lives with the wisdom they have preserved.

Seasonal and Local Eating

The Hadzabe source their meals directly from their environment, relying on the bounty of each season to dictate what's on the menu. From tubers and fruits to fresh-caught game, their diet is a dance with nature, evolving as seasons change. This harmony with what the land provides is a testament to the benefits of eating local and seasonal food.

The Hadzabes' way of eating is a vibrant reminder of how our ancestors lived in tune with the earth's natural cycles. This starkly contrasts with our modern convenience-driven habits, where strawberries are perpetually in season, and asparagus is available year-round, often shipped from faraway lands. While global accessibility is undoubtedly compelling, our deviation from seasonal eating comes at a cost.

Research reveals that consuming fresh produce from the season enhances nutrient availability. Take a strawberry picked at its ripest; it's not just brimming with flavor, it's bursting with nutrients. Seasonal eating ensures that fruits and vegetables are consumed when their nutritional content peaks, offering us more vitamins and minerals than their out-of-season counterparts, often harvested prematurely and artificially ripened.

We support our health, local farms, and ecosystems by focusing on local produce. Eating locally is also environmentally friendly, reducing the carbon footprint associated with long-distance transport. Moreover, local produce often contains fewer preservatives and chemicals, preserving its purity and reducing exposure to potentially harmful substances.

Aligning our diet with what's in season also complements our bodies' natural circadian rhythms. Consuming seasonal and local foods can enhance physical harmony by providing nutrients suited to each season's specific climate and energy requirements. In warmer months, lighter fruits and vegetables hydrate and refresh, while denser, starchy foods offer warmth and sustenance in colder times.

Modern science underscores how eating harmoniously with the seasons may improve health and well-being. For instance, winter squash contains higher levels of vitamins A and C needed for immune function, aligning well with the months when colds are prevalent. Meanwhile, summer tomatoes are rich in antioxidants that offer some protection against the effects of prolonged sun exposure.

While technology has revolutionized our access to food, there's much to gain by reviving the primal ways, from reconnecting with nature's rhythm and supporting local bounty to optimizing nutrition by aligning our diet with each passing season.

Connection to Nature and Mindful Eating

As we move forward from seasonal and local foods, let's delve into the remarkable relationship the Hadzabe nurture with the natural world, a bond steeped in an intuitive understanding of food sourcing and consumption, a page of history that offers us an inspiring lesson in mindful eating.

Picture the Hadzabe in their lush Tanzanian habitat, where food isn't just nourishment, it's a vital thread in the tapestry of life. Every meal is a hands-on affair rooted in the natural environment. Whether hunting game with hand-crafted bows or foraging for berries and wild tubers, the Hadzabe embody a profound connection with their food sources. In this context, eating is more than survival; it's a dance with nature, a reciprocal partnership where the earth provides, and gratitude is the unspoken currency.

Contrast this harmonious dynamic with our modern food systems. Today, the convenience of pre-packaged, processed foods has distanced many of us from the origins of our meals. When shopping in supermarkets, we often forget the journey of food to reach our plates. This disconnection can lead to overconsumption and waste, as there's little sense of the energy and effort that's gone into food production.

Reconnecting with our food sources calls for a mindful approach to eating. Mindful eating is about slowing down, tuning into hunger cues, savoring flavors and textures, and genuinely appreciating the meal before us. This practice enhances our eating experience and aligns our physical and mental well-being with the nourishment we receive.

Research supports the psychological benefits of mindfulness in eating. Studies have shown that attention to our hunger signals and eating can improve digestion, reduce stress, and help prevent overeating. Mindful eating encourages awareness of the body's needs, ushering us away from mindless snacking and emotional eating.

By forging a genuine bond with our food and practicing mindful eating, we can echo the Hadzabes' respect for nature, fostering a profound connection to the world around us. In doing so, we nurture a balanced approach to food and health that aligns with nature's enduring wisdom.

Nutrient Density versus Caloric Density

Imagine straying from a world bombarded by processed temptations to sit by a campfire with the Hadzabe tribe, where meals aren't just about taste but about life itself. In their corner of the world, food remains a daily celebration of nutrient density, a concept too often overshadowed by our love affair with hyper-palatable offerings.

The Hadzabe thrive on a diet emphasizing high-nutrient, low-calorie foods, serving up a smorgasbord rich in essential vitamins and minerals. Their meals are master classes in nutrition. Everything they consume, from protein-packed bugs to vibrant berries, ensures balanced nutrition without overloading calories.

Unlike those of us who navigate urban supermarkets stacked with sizzle, their primary goal isn't to tempt taste buds but to nourish body and soul while warding off metabolic mischief makers like obesity and type 2 diabetes. Studies highlight that nutrient-dense diets can lower the risks of developing such diseases while offering a natural supplementation of vitamins and minerals that modern supplements can only hope to mimic.

Now, let's detour to our world, where food manufacturers are engaged in an ongoing quest to engineer flavors that seduce our senses. Hyperpalatable foods are a wolf in sheep's clothing; they pack a walloping calorie punch while disguising their lack of nutritional clout. Think about those midnight snack runs that end in a frenzy of guilt and a little extra "fluff" around the waist.

Modern diets rich in such calorie-dense and nutrient-poor foods correlate with a spike in chronic diseases, draining health while filling plates with temptation. These foods fuel obesity and diabetes while keeping us sated on empty promises.

Returning to nutrient-dense foods isn't about compromise; it's about choosing to nourish, replenish, and energize through mindful eating rooted in age-old traditions. By portioning our plates with vegetables, fruits, lean proteins, and whole grains, we mirror the Hadzabes' wisdom, their konwing that food is sustenance, strength, and song.

Let your next meal be a testament to vitality. Swap hyperpalatable treats for fruits that paint your tongue with poetry or vegetables that crunch like a symphony. We were never meant for a diet of empty echoes; we were designed for the richness of life.

Digging Deep: The Issue of Soil Depletion and Nutrient Density

As we step from the vibrant world of nutrient density into the gritty realities of soil health, it becomes clear that our food's nutritional power begins long before it reaches our plates, right at the soil it's grown in. If we're serious about transforming our diets, we must grasp the profound relationship between the earth and what it yields.

Imagine wandering through the lush landscapes of an African savanna, where the soil is rich and fertile, teeming with life and nutrients. This vibrant earth fuels the plants, which, in turn, nourish the wildlife and the people nearby. In these pristine environments, the food harvested is inherently superior, bursting with flavors and essential nutrients. Unfortunately, this is not the story for many farmed foods in the modern agricultural landscape.

Soil depletion is more than just an environmental buzzword; it's a pressing crisis threatening our food systems and overall health. **According to the UN Food and Agriculture Organization (FAO), approximately one-third of the world's soils are currently considered to be degraded, and over 90% could become degraded by 2050.** This is primarily due to intensive agricultural practices, deforestation, and urbanization. A staggering 75 billion tons of fertile soil is lost each year, due to erosion. We are losing the foundation of our food sources.

Moreover, soil nutrient depletion is evidenced by the declining nutrient profiles of commonly consumed crops. Between 1950 and the early 2000s, many fruits, vegetables, and grains declined in essential nutrients such as vitamins and minerals due to lackluster soil health and agricultural inputs. We may be eating more, but our plates are less nourishing.

The difference between the nutrient-packed foods from fertile soils in tribal regions and the often diminished, nutritionally hollow produce from modern farms is stark. Research has shown that crop nutrient levels can significantly vary based on soil health and farming practices, resulting in foods that fail to deliver the vitamins and minerals essential for optimal health. We can practically taste the difference—and feel the effects.

In places like the African savanna, where soil has developed over millennia in a symbiotic relationship with the flora and fauna, you find a rich tapestry of nutrients essential for sustaining vibrant ecosystems. Here, organic matter nurtures a diverse microbial life in the soil, leading to increased fertility that, in turn, cultivates crops bursting with vitamins, minerals, and antioxidants. Conversely, modern agricultural practices often strip soils of these critical elements, creating a cycle of depletion that robs our food of its integrity.

Amidst these alarming statistics, one cannot help but wonder: What can we do about it? Reconnecting with our food sources is paramount. Seek out local farms that practice sustainable agriculture, where crop rotation, diverse planting, and natural fertilization techniques breathe new life into the soil. In doing so, you will enjoy tastier produce and support methods that restore the soil's natural fertility.

This awareness transcends individual choices; backing regenerative agriculture fosters healthier ecosystems that produce nutrient-dense foods, ultimately bolstering our communal health. As we navigate the delicate balance between soil health and nutritional density, let's remember that the earth is not only our provider but also our partner in health.

Primal Living and Mitochondrial Health

Picture this: Deep within your cells are tiny power plants, known as mitochondria, working tirelessly to keep you moving and grooving. These little dynamos convert food into energy, fueling every heartbeat, breath, and thought. Yet in the modern world, with its conveniences and processed foods, we often overlook or sabotage these cellular engines. Could we learn a lesson or two from the African tribal cultures, who seem to have cracked the code of mitochondrial optimization?

Mitochondria are the unsung heroes within our cells. They produce adenosine triphosphate (ATP), the primary energy currency that powers cellular functions. Think of ATP as the high-octane fuel driving your bodily Ferrari; when mitochondria work efficiently, we feel energetic and vibrant. But when they falter, we experience fatigue, cognitive sluggishness, and a general decline in health.

African tribal cultures, with their natural lifestyles and nutrient-rich diets, tend to support robust mitochondrial function. Regular physical activity and diets high in antioxidants and healthy fats (think omega-3s from wild game and essential nutrients from vibrant fruits and vegetables) bolster mitochondrial efficiency.

Contrastingly, our modern lifestyles can undermine these cellular powerhouses. Diets heavy in processed foods, loaded with sugars and unhealthy fats, contribute to oxidative stress, damaging mitochondria. A sedentary lifestyle can further exacerbate mitochondrial decline, reducing their capacity to generate sufficient energy. The research underscores the role of oxidative stress in mitochondrial damage.

African tribal practices showcase how natural living supports vibrant health. By embracing the same ethos in our lives, we can harness the power of our mitochondria, fueling our bodies and minds with boundless energy and vigor.

Reviving Cellular Powerhouses: Mitochondria in the Modern Age

The trappings of modern life can stifle mitochondrial effectiveness, altering processes critical to our health, such as mitochondrial biogenesis, mitochondrial dynamics, and mitophagy. To truly understand how contemporary lifestyles impact these processes, we must delve into each concept's importance and reflect on how ancestral lifestyles, like those of the Hadzabe, promote optimal mitochondrial health.

Mitochondrial Biogenesis: Building More Power Plants

Mitochondrial biogenesis is the process of forming new mitochondria within a cell, critical for maintaining energy production and cellular function. Our activity levels and diet significantly influence this process. Regular physical exercise and intermittent fasting are well-documented promoters of mitochondrial biogenesis. They initiate cellular signals that ramp up the production of new mitochondria, enhancing energy capacity and endurance.

Modern sedentary lifestyles and poor dietary habits provide little incentive for mitochondrial biogenesis. Sedentary lifestyles lead to decreased energy needs, resulting in fewer mitochondria and lower cellular efficiency. In contrast, the Hadzabes' way of life, which is characterized by continual physical movement and reliance on natural, nutrient-rich foods, aligns more closely with conditions that foster mitochondrial growth and vitality.

Mitochondrial Dynamics: The Ballet of Fission and Fusion

Mitochondrial dynamics refers to the balance of fission (splitting) and fusion (joining) events that allow mitochondria to adapt to a cell's changing energy demands. This dynamic balance is crucial for maintaining mitochondrial function and distribution within cells. In healthy circumstances, mitochondria can fuse to efficiently share resources and genetic material, while fission allows damaged mitochondria to be segregated for degradation.

The hectic pace of modern life, with chronic stress and inconsistent sleep patterns, can disrupt this finely tuned dance, leading to mitochondrial dysfunction. Stress-induced signaling pathways can alter the delicate interplay of fission and fusion, impairing energy metabolism and contributing to health issues. The Hadzabe, with a lifestyle rooted in a harmonious rhythm that includes natural cycles of activity and rest, probably experience optimal mitochondrial dynamics, bolstering their resilience against oxidative stress.

Mitophagy: The Cleansing Ritual

Mitophagy is the selective degradation of damaged mitochondria, akin to a cellular cleansing ritual, that ensures only the healthiest mitochondria persist. This process is vital for preventing the accumulation of dysfunctional mitochondria that can lead to cellular damage and age-related diseases.

Our modern environment, characterized by exposure to pollutants, excess caloric intake, and lack of exercise, burdens mitophagy. An overabundance of damaged mitochondria impairs cellular health and accelerates aging. In contrast, the Hadzabes' lifestyle, with its natural fasting periods between meals and physically demanding daily activities, likely enhances mitophagy, facilitating cellular renewal and protection.

Primal Insights for Mitochondrial Health

To draw upon the wisdom of our ancestors and foster mitochondrial health, consider integrating the following primal practices into your modern life:

1. **Rigorous Physical Activity:** Engage in daily activities that mirror the Hadzabes' physical lifestyle: walking, running, and climbing. Exercise stimulates mitochondrial biogenesis, enhancing energy production.

2. **Balanced Diet with Fasting:** Incorporate intermittent fasting and nutrient-dense foods, similar to the Hadzabes' foraging diet, to promote mitophagy and optimize mitochondrial function.

3. **Stress Management and Rest:** Embrace stress-reduction techniques and prioritize restful sleep to support mitochondrial dynamics and resilience against modern stressors.

By understanding and nurturing these mitochondrial processes, we can align our lifestyles with those that sustain health and vitality over generations. Learning from the Hadzabe, we appreciate the power of movement, nourishment, and balance in fostering robust cellular energetics, lessons that are just as relevant today as they have been throughout human history.

Sugar and Refined Carbohydrates—A Modern Epidemic

Stroll down the aisles of any supermarket, and you'll find a veritable field of sugary temptations, each product promising a sweet escape. From cereals and sodas to sauces and snacks, added sugars have been stealthily woven into our modern diet's fabric. But while these sugary delights may offer a temporary high, they come with long-term costs that are anything but sweet.

In stark contrast, primal diets, reminiscent of those consumed by our hunter-gatherer ancestors, were virtually devoid of refined sugars. Instead, their sweetness came naturally from honey or the occasional ripe fruit sparingly consumed due to the effort required in obtaining it. This natural, minimal sugar intake aligns with a lifestyle where obesity, diabetes, and metabolic syndrome are virtually nonexistent.

Modern diets, however, have embraced sugar with open arms and extended waistlines. The ubiquity of refined sugars and carbohydrates in our food supply is not optional; it's pervasive, contributing to a surge in chronic diseases. Estimates suggest that the average American consumes about **17 teaspoons**

of added sugar per day, a stark contrast to the American Heart Association's recommendation of just **6 teaspoons for women and 9 teaspoons for men.**

Refined carbohydrates, particularly sugars, have profound effects on our health. Research has linked these dietary staples to chronic inflammation, insulin resistance, and fat accumulation, the trifecta behind many modern health woes. Studies highlight how refined carbs cause rapid spikes and drops in blood sugar, a rollercoaster that not only sends hunger signals into overdrive but also fosters an environment ripe for metabolic dysfunction.

Moreover, these rapid fluctuations in glucose levels burden the pancreas with insulin overproduction, eventually leading to insulin resistance. In this condition, the body's cells become less responsive to insulin, forcing blood sugar levels to climb. This relentless cycle is a key player in the development of type 2 diabetes and can accelerate fat storage, contributing to obesity and chronic health issues.

By mirroring the wisdom of primal diets and respecting the evolutionary blueprint, we can mitigate the impact of refined carbs and sugars, paving the way for improved health and vitality. As modern science affirms, the less sugar we consume, the sweeter our health outcomes will likely be.

Epigenetics and Nutrition: The Symphony Between Food and Our Genes

In the fascinating arena of epigenetics, our DNA may have the music sheets, but the epigenetic markers conduct the symphony, dictating the performance of our genes. While we're given a genetic blueprint at birth, lifestyle choices often play the role of maestro, influencing which genes take center stage and which remain silent in the background. Among these lifestyle choices, nutrition emerges as a powerful baton capable of orchestrating our health and longevity.

Imagine your genes as the intricate keys of a grand piano. The activation of epigenetic factors can strike a melodious harmony or discordant notes, affecting everything from longevity to disease susceptibility. The foods we consume provide the notes and rhythm to this composition through molecules that interact with our genes and help fine-tune their expression.

Diet can activate or silence genes through DNA methylation and histone modification. Certain nutrients found in food can promote DNA methylation, attaching methyl groups to specific DNA segments to silence genes that promote inflammation or cancer. Similarly, histone modifications can lead to tighter or looser DNA packing around histone proteins, impacting gene accessibility and expression.

Foods rich in bioactive compounds, such as green tea, turmeric, and cruciferous vegetables, contain potent epigenetic modulators that can switch off oncogenes or activate tumor suppressor genes. These dietary elements act like conductors, modulating the notes played by our genes, thereby affecting our risk factors for various age-related diseases.

Primal Diets and Epigenetic Signaling

When examining the impact of nutrition on genetics, it's helpful to consider primal diets rich in whole foods, natural fats, lean proteins, and fibrous carbohydrates. These diets have long supported optimal human health by influencing gene activity. Primal diets are rich in nutrients and phytochemicals that support healthy epigenetic modifications, promoting longevity and robust health.

Our ancient ancestors' diets, high in omega-3 fatty acids, antioxidants, and myriad micronutrients, encouraged beneficial epigenetic changes that favored inflammation reduction and immune regulation. The absence of processed foods and excess sugars minimized detrimental gene activations, nature's way of protecting our biological heritage.

While modern diets have introduced new challenges with processed ingredients, the principles of a primal diet emphasize a return to these epigenetically beneficial foods. Nutrient-dense items from this dietary repertoire can help maintain optimal gene expression and better regulate biological pathways associated with aging and disease.

Harnessing the power of nutrition means mindfully choosing what we consume and recognizing its potential to script our genetic narrative. By adopting a diet rich in whole, unprocessed foods, we can achieve optimal genetic expression, promoting longevity, reducing disease risk, and enhancing our overall health. With each meal, we take charge, orchestrating a symphony where our genes perform their intended roles in harmony and wellness. Let us savor nature's bounty, understanding that every bite resonates through our DNA, shaping a life of health and balance.

Our Connection with Food

As we wrap up our exploration of the nourishing bonds we form with food, it's time to tackle the ultimate question: Does the food we shovel into our mouths give us life, or does it drain us of energy? The Hadzabe don't follow a diet or rigid rules about what's edible and what's not. Instead, they understand what keeps them vigorous and vibrant, grounded in their direct connection with nature.

Food: Life-Promoting vs. Life-Depleting

In many Eastern cultures, food isn't just for filling bellies; it's a source of life force, known as prana or chi. Foods are seen as either supporting this life force or detracting from it. Ayurveda takes this philosophy a step further, classifying foods into Sattvic, Rajasic, and Tamasic categories based on the energy and physiological effects they impart.

Satvic Foods: Nurturers of Life

Satvic foods are the crème de la crème of the Ayurvedic diet, bursting with pure, fresh ingredients that promote vitality. Imagine colorful vegetables, whole grains, nutty snacks, and ripe fruits, all harvested at their peak and ready to nourish the body, mind, and spirit. Scientific research backs up the benefits of these foods, linking whole-food diets with better health outcomes, reduced inflammation, and enhanced mental well-being. Consuming Satvic foods sets the stage for a vibrant life, creating an internal environment where health flourishes.

Rajasic Foods: The Energizers

Now, let's turn our attention to Rajasic foods, the spirited side of the culinary spectrum. These foods (think spicy dishes, caffeinated drinks, and hearty fare) are known for revving the body and mind. While they can ignite energy and creativity, too much zest can lead to jitters and restlessness, like downing that double espresso that kicks your day into high gear but leaves you crashing later. Moderation is key, so balance Rajasic choices with Satvic foods to keep the body in harmony. After all, life is all about the right mix!

Tamasic Foods: The Weighty Choices

On the flip side are Tamasic foods, those that are stale, overly processed, and lacking in substance. These choices can drain your energy rather than replenish it. Think of them as the couch potato of your diet, lulling you into lethargy when you need a boost. These foods contribute to modern ailments, adversely affecting our health and vitality.

While traditional African tribal cultures like the Hadzabe may not have categorized their foods using Ayurvedic terms, their intuitive choices make it clear that they gravitate toward what nourishes and lifts their spirits. Their diets are full of whole, unprocessed foods rich in nutrition and deeply connected to their environment.

The bridge connecting ancient wisdom with contemporary science reveals a profound relationship with food that many of us can reclaim. Diets rich in nutrient-dense foods positively impact our health markers, metabolic function, and energy levels. Conversely, the negative effects of Tamasic foods resonate with the alarming rise in chronic conditions that haunt modern society, reminding us that our food choices shape our health destiny. Life-depleting foods throw a wrench into our finely tuned biological machinery. They stoke inflammation, raise heart rates, and leave us feeling more like a used dishrag than the robust beings we ought to be.

A Simple Test

Want a quick way to gauge how a particular food affects you? Check your heart rate after eating. Foods that disagree with us often raise our heart rates, signaling the internal army to prepare for battle rather than peaceful assimilation. It's your body waving a red flag, asking for culinary betterment.

We must remember our bodies are born from the earth. Water makes up about 70% of both the planet's surface and our physical composition. Foods that stay truest to this origin align harmoniously with our bodies, making digestion a breeze rather than a burden. The closer our food sources are to the earth's own, the simpler they are for us to process.

As a general rule, strive for a diet where 80% of your food is unprocessed and close to its natural state. Think whole grains over white bread, fresh fruit over fruit juice, and dark leafy greens that look like they were plucked from the garden that morning. It's about returning to that innate wisdom so many of us have lost, like the Hadzabe, who understand food as a source of vitality rather than a mere commodity.

Reflecting on Our Journey

Through this chapter on nourishing bonds, we've woven together knowledge from ancient practices and modern science, all in pursuit of a healthier, more connected relationship with what we eat. Whether you're reaching for a vibrant salad, rich in color and life, or an indulgent dish slathered in sauces and conveniences, remember the choices we make not only feed our hunger but define our connection to the world we inhabit.

Our forebears intuitively understood how their bodies responded to what they consumed. By consciously integrating these principles into our modern lives, we can cultivate nourishing relationships with food that promote vitality and well-being.

As we bid farewell to this chapter, let it serve as a guidepost—not a strict set of rules but an invitation to engage passionately and mindfully with our food, forging connections that sustain not just our bodies but our communities, our environments, and the eternal dance of life itself. So, here's to eating well, living richly, and celebrating the bonds that nourish and unite us all.

Primal Practices:

1. Gradual Intermittent Fasting:

Start extending the time between dinner and breakfast gradually, moving toward the 16/8 method, where you fast for 16 hours and eat within an 8-hour window. This method helps your body adapt and can enhance metabolic health while you stay hydrated and savor each meal.

2. Mindful Movement During Fasting:

Include light physical activities like walking or stretching during fasting periods to boost fat burning and support metabolism without overwhelming the body.

3. Embrace Fiber:

Regularly consume a variety of fiber-rich foods, such as fruits, vegetables, legumes, and whole grains, to enhance gut health and support a diverse microbiome.

4. Incorporate Fermented Foods:

Add fermented items like yogurt, kefir, kimchi, and sauerkraut to your meals, introducing beneficial probiotics that nourish your gut bacteria.

5. Support Local and Seasonal Eating:

Visit farmers' markets to explore fresh, seasonal produce while supporting local agriculture. Join a Community Supported Agriculture (CSA) program. Advocate for and support local farmers and food systems prioritizing regenerative agricultural practices. Let the seasons guide your culinary adventures with fresh and vibrant ingredients.

6. Color Your Meals:

Fill your plate with colorful vegetables and fruits for a diverse intake of essential nutrients. Aim for various colors at every meal, treating your plate as a canvas of health.

7. Mindful Eating Practices:

Focus on eating without distractions, savoring the flavors, colors, and textures, and tuning into your hunger signals to prevent overeating.

8. Limit Sugar and Processed Foods:

Opt for whole, unprocessed foods rich in natural fiber and nutrients instead of calorie-dense snacks. This practice reduces the risk of metabolic disorders and promotes long-term health.

9. Cultivate a Connection with Food Sources:

Spend time understanding where your food comes from, starting a small garden, or engaging with local food systems to build a connection to the earth.

10. Prioritize Antioxidant-Rich and Healthy Fat Foods:

Incorporate foods rich in antioxidants and omega-3s, such as berries, leafy greens, and fish, to support mitochondrial health and overall energy production.

4

MINDFUL UNITY: CULTIVATING THE MIND-BODY CONNECTION

"The mind and body are not separate.
What affects one, affects the other."
– Anonymous

A Journey from the Savanna to Silence

The vastness of the African savanna unfolded before my eyes like a never-ending tapestry of golden grasses and distant horizons. As a child, I remember watching a Hadzabe hunter standing at the edge of this breathtaking expanse. He was the embodiment of stillness. His eyes, steady and piercing, seemed to lock onto the horizon as if deciphering a secret only known to the ancients. In that moment, time paused. There was nothing to do, nowhere to go. It was as if the quiet enveloped him, forming his mind and body into a serene unity.

I often wondered what thoughts occupied his mind, if any at all. Was there a vibrant symphony of life playing in the recesses of his being? Or was it merely emptiness, an undisturbed pool reflecting the savanna's glory? It wasn't until many years later, when I reached my forties and found myself uncomfortably disconnected, that I would begin to uncover the mysteries behind those eyes.

In the bustle of adult life, I craved the harmony and presence that the hunter embodied. This yearning led me to explore contemplative practices designed to bridge the gap between mind and body. My pursuit eventually brought me to an eight-day silent retreat focused on the art of breath-watching. The experience was anything but serene at first; the incessant chatter of my mind echoed like a clamor of discordant instruments, and frustration danced closely, tempting me to call it quits.

For six days, I grappled with my inner chatter. Each session felt like a battle of wills: my racing thoughts against my yearning for peace. But on day seven, exhaustion overtook frustration. I had no energy to resist or be frustrated. I simply let go. As I surrendered to the process, my breath became rhythmic, unforced. In that moment, I'd begun to mirror the Hadzabes' grace.

Then it happened. As I sat there, eyes softly opened, my thoughts dropped away, revealing the profound silence beneath. There was no yesterday or tomorrow, no chaos of modern life blinking in the background. Time seemed to hold its breath. In an instant, I was transported back to my childhood in the savanna, reliving the stillness of the Hadzabe hunter. I realized that he had been unconsciously practicing a form of standing meditation with eyes wide open, innately connected to his environment and self.

I understood, at last, that meditation isn't merely a practice, it's a homecoming. It's a return to a state of unity and calm that we instinctively yearn for. In our attempts to escape the relentless monkey chatter of our minds, we often turn to distractions like alcohol, drugs, or extreme sports, searching for the fleeting moments when time and thought cease. Yet the stillness I found required none of these crutches, only the embrace of conscious presence.

In this chapter, we explore the profound unity between mind and body. We delve into practices that harmonize these two realms, fostering improved biological age and longevity. Examining facets of stillness through scientific and ancient lenses, our journey will reveal how the frantic dance of the mind can be tamed. Like the Hadzabe hunter, we'll discover how to cultivate enduring peace, finding tranquility beneath life's ever-present winds.

"Chitta Vritti Nirodhah"

Centuries ago, an exceptional yogi dedicated himself to exploring the entire human mechanism in order to achieve ultimate health for humanity. After thoroughly examining everything, he distilled his insights into three words: "Chitta Vritti Nirodhah," which means calming the fluctuations of the mind. This yogi, Patanjali, often referred to as the father of yoga, believed that this principle held the key to alleviating all human suffering.

Mind: The Ever-Shaken Snowglobe

Imagine, if you will, your mind as a snow globe. In our routines, we become habitual shakers of this globe. Each flurry of thoughts, all the anxieties about tomorrow, and the regrets of yesterday cloud the clarity of our present moment. The snowflakes, those endless thoughts and worries, obscure our ability to perceive reality as it is. We project our fears and insecurities onto our world, never allowing the snow to settle, never resting in the here and now.

In our modern society, we often lead fragmented lives. Our minds are consumed by regrets from the past or worries about the future, while our bodies operate without conscious awareness. This disconnect can contribute to chronic stress and various health issues. Our body's stress response was designed for short bursts, for escaping lions, not day-long marathons of emails and existential angst. When stress becomes our default mode, our health pays the price, impacting everything from our cardiovascular system to our overall resilience.

Stress and Cortisol in Aging

We all intuitively know that stress accelerates the aging process. Yet, in our fast-paced lives, stress seems inescapable. This isn't just an unwanted emotion but a major player governing our biology.

Stress has an evolutionary origin rooted in our survival mechanism. When faced with danger, the immediate surge of adrenaline and cortisol is key to recruiting the mental and physical resources to fight or flee. This primal design was critical when encountering lions in the wild; however, we are rarely confronted with such dangers in the modern world. **The most interesting phenomenon is that in today's world, we have a multitude of "micro-lions" in the form of deadlines, bills, and buzzing smartphones that have replaced the original predators, with the same biological consequences.** While encounters with actual lions were rare and necessitated an acute stress response, the "micro-lions" are all around us and lead to a state of chronic stress, with constantly elevated cortisol levels negatively impacting our bodies.

Cortisol, commonly known as the stress hormone, plays a crucial role in our fight-or-flight response. When cortisol is chronically elevated due to prolonged stress, it can adversely impact our health. One key biological mechanism affected by this process is telomere shortening. Telomeres are protective caps at the end of our chromosomes and play a role in maintaining genomic stability. Chronic stress leads to telomere shortening and can potentially accelerate cellular aging, increasing the risk of age-related diseases such as diabetes, cardiovascular disease, and immune dysfunction.

Radiologist's Revelation: Seeing the Mind-Body Link

The dimly lit radiology room, with the gentle hum of the computer fan and the soft glow of the computer screen, has an almost Zen-like atmosphere (most of my friends wonder how I stay awake). What keeps me alert is the story each scan on the screen holds. I tell people they can lie to me all they want, but their bodies will always tell the truth on my screen. Yet our physical body is only half the equation. What I don't see, and always wonder about, is the kind of mind that led to the body I see in front of me. There is an intricate dance between our physical health and emotional well-being.

I often encounter a fascinating paradox that never fails to capture my curiosity. As a neuroradiologist, I often try to guess the patient's age based on the level of volume loss in the brain. I am frequently surprised by an 80-year-old with the brain size of someone half his age. Conversely, it's shocking to see a young patient whose brain suggests atrophy as though the years have prematurely aged this person.

What's the octogenarian's secret to preserving brain health? Has this individual tapped into some primal intelligence of cognitive vitality? I imagine them navigating and riding life's waves with mindful resilience, agility, and thoughtful spirit.

In neuroscience, this mechanism of mental vitality is best understood from the framework of neuroplasticity, which is the brain's ability to mold itself, reorganize, and regenerate through life's experiences. Imagine the brain as a lush Amazon rainforest with a unique ecosystem containing areas of new growth and regions of decay. Specific neural pathways, like forest footpaths, become more established with frequent use, while others wither away due to neglect. This capacity for renewal and growth is at the heart of what keeps our minds young, agile, and responsive, regardless of age.

Our primal intelligence has equipped us to nurture this delicate ecosystem. Primitive tribes like the Hadzabe don't just survive; they thrive by constantly adapting to ever-changing environments, engaging in social interactions, and tackling daily challenges like hunting. This intrinsic adaptability is ingrained in our ancestral DNA and continues to influence our synapses (neuronal connections) today. Our primal design calls us to stay physically active, intellectually curious, and socially connected.

The 80-year-old with the "young" brain is undoubtedly engaged in a lifestyle promoting physical activity, continuous learning, and social engagement, cultivating neural expansion and resilience. Research supports this observation, showing that problem-solving, exercise, and socialization significantly impact brain health. These "brain workouts" strengthen synaptic connections and stave off cognitive decline, allowing the mind to remain nimble and vibrant.

Remarkably, neuroplasticity works in reverse as well. When we neglect our primal imperative to engage with our environment and challenge ourselves, the brain mirrors our sedentary life no matter our chronological age. It's a dynamic reflection of our mind-body connection. Every time I notice an unexpected discrepancy in biological and chronological age on my scans, I'm reminded of our lifestyle choices' sheer power in molding us. The key lies in engaging with the world, seizing opportunities to learn, adapt, and connect, nourishing our cerebral ecosystem.

**Age is just a number, but vitality is a testament
to how we choose to live.**

Rewiring Youth: The Neuroplasticity of Mindful Living

The human brain's primal ability to rewire and regenerate is its superpower and the key to longevity. Contemplative practices like meditation fine-tune our mind-body connection, enhance neuroplasticity, and surprisingly reverse bio-logical aging.

Mindfulness Meditation: The Brain's Personal Trainer

Mindfulness meditation stands out among the contemplative practices with many brain health benefits. Studies have used functional MRI scans to reveal that reg-ular mindfulness meditation increased cortical thickness in the prefrontal cor-tex, which is responsible for decision-making, focus, and emotional regulation while shrinking the stress-harboring amygdala region of the brain. Meditation isn't just a relaxing activity, it is brain-sculpting! The reported increased cortical thickness observed in the minds of meditators correlates with improved mem-ory and emotional steadiness. It's like upgrading your central nervous system hardware, improving performance and efficiency.

Slowing Brain Aging: Pressing Pause on the Biological Clock

The most inspiring findings come from studies on long-term meditators who demonstrated brains remarkably younger than their chronological age might suggest. Meditation preserved gray matter volume and acted as a neuroprotective agent against the cognitive decline often seen with old age. What if your mindfulness practice could serve as a pause button on your brain's biological clock? While these findings don't offer immortality, they highlight our built-in primal mechanisms to maintain cognitive health.

Mindfulness meditation is a life-enhancing neuro hack. When you meditate, you engage in a mental workout that targets neuroplasticity and cultivates a youthful brain. Those quiet moments on the meditation cushion allow us to find peace and a scientifically backed path toward longevity and cognitive vitality.

Stillness versus Illness: A Journey Toward Inner Harmony

In today's world, stillness is a rare commodity. It is no wonder Patanjali mentioned that the ultimate remedy is "chitta vritti nirodha," calming the mind's disturbances. When we find stillness, we experience a sense of ease; where there is **ease**, there is no **DISease**. Therefore, the ultimate choice is between stillness and illness.

A core component of cultivating stillness is understanding our parasympathetic nervous system, which serves as the body's natural mechanism for rest and repair. Think of it as a spa retreat for your nervous system, promoting relaxation and restoration. This starkly contrasts with the sympathetic "fight or flight" mode that modern life constantly keeps us in.

In a sympathetic state, cortisol (our stress hormone) levels rise, and energy reserves become depleted. When we are anxious, we feel drained and exhausted. This is partly because **our brains, which account for just 2% of our body weight, consume 20% of our total energy.** Functional MRI imaging shows that our brain energy demands significantly decrease during restful states. This allows for cellular repair and mental rejuvenation.

However, this state of rest remains elusive without intentional efforts to cultivate stillness. Instead, we find ourselves on a perpetual treadmill, chasing deadlines and digital notifications while the promise of tranquility slips further away. Each ping nudges us toward a state of perpetual alertness. It's as though we have invited chaos into our pockets, robbing us of our stillness every time we check our devices.

While social media platforms promise connection, they can also pull us away from the present moment. They engross us in curated realities, leading us to Comparison Ville, where everyone's life seems more exciting or successful than our own. This focus on external validation disrupts our peace and leaves us vulnerable to anxiety and dissatisfaction.

Choosing stillness is a conscious decision to prioritize well-being over chronic stress. When we create internal harmony, we reduce disease risk and enhance life satisfaction. Stillness allows us to embrace the moment. Health isn't just about the absence of illness but the presence of tranquility. The journey to stillness in a frantic world begins with paying attention to simple things like our breath.

Anapanasati Yoga: The Art of Breath Awareness

The term "anapanasati" comes from two Sanskrit words: "anapana," which means "in-breath" and "out-breath," and "sati," which means "awareness" or "mindfulness." This ancient technique, which dates back over two thousand years, provides a pathway to profound awareness through the focused practice of breath. Its origins can be traced back to ancient Buddhist texts that outline the foundations of mindfulness practice.

Anapanasati is more than just a meditation technique; it uses the breath as a bridge to connect the body and mind. The Buddha emphasized breath-watching as a means of achieving greater insight and tranquility. Through this practice, individuals learn to anchor themselves in the present moment by observing their breath as it flows naturally. The key is not to control the breath; one should allow it to happen naturally. **In a time when the desire for control often leads to stress, this act of surrender becomes a transformative gift.**

The core principle of Anapanasati Yoga is conscious breathing. Our pattern and depth of inhalation and exhalation reflect our inner state of being. The goal is not to alter our breath but to cultivate an open and receptive awareness of the sensations that arise with each inhalation and exhalation. This practice may seem simple, but it is incredibly powerful and can transform our mental status.

Research supports the significant impact of breath awareness on our physiological and psychological states. Breathing-focused practices have been linked to reduced stress levels, improved emotional regulation, and enhanced cognitive function. By consciously directing our attention to our breath, we activate the parasympathetic nervous system, our body's natural pathway to relaxation.

Monkey Mind: Taming the Wandering Thoughts

Yet, as anyone who has attempted Anapanasati will attest, this seemingly straightforward practice comes with its challenges. Each time you settle into your practice, your mind may insist on some adventure, such as recalling undone tasks, daydreaming about future plans, or revisiting past conversations. This is the nature of the mind; it tends to wander, veering away from the simple, present act of breathing. The term "monkey mind" aptly captures the frantic nature of our wandering thoughts.

Functional MRI imaging of the wandering mind demonstrates the activation of the Default Mode Network (DMN). The DMN is a network of brain regions that shows increased activity when we are at rest and not focused on the outside world or involved in an active task. It is active when we daydream, reminisce, or let our minds wander. It's like the brain's background music playing when we aren't directly engaged in a task.

Interestingly, rather than experiencing calming thoughts during moments of downtime, our minds often dive into turbulent waters. Instead of basking in tranquility, the DMN pulls us into the murky depths of past regrets and future anxieties, expertly luring us away from stillness. Conversely, while we once thought downtime meant relaxation, it can inadvertently lead us into a mental cyclone, an uninvited dip back into the chaos of life's stressors.

The irony is that we often find ourselves caught in a web of overthinking when we pursue calmness. The more we wish to quiet our minds, the more agitated they become. This dance of thoughts challenges our understanding of mental health. How can we reclaim our minds amidst such chaos?

It's in this acknowledgment, the embrace of your mind's tendencies, that the real power of Anapanasati emerges. **Rather than engaging in a battle**

against your wandering thoughts, you cultivate the skill of gently redirecting your focus back to your breath. This act of returning is where mindfulness flourishes. Every time you guide your attention back when it has strayed, you're flexing the "muscle" of mindfulness, enhancing your ability to remain present in all aspects of life. Observing our wandering minds creates space between ourselves and our thoughts, allowing us to return to a state of stillness and clarity.

The simple act of breathing offers the opportunity for profound transformation. We reconnect with ourselves with every inhalation and exhalation, bridging the gap between the mind and body in delightful harmony. Ultimately, the journey from monkey mind to mindful living is an ongoing endeavor.

Breath as the Bridge: Pranayama and Longevity

You can follow the cleanest diet, lift weights, and take every anti-aging supplement available, but if your breathing is dysfunctional, your longevity is at risk. Breathing isn't just about taking in oxygen; it's about life force, nervous system control, and metabolic efficiency. Unfortunately, in the modern world, we often breathe too quickly, too shallowly, and too chaotically, living in a state of low-grade panic and unaware that our breath is a remote control governing our biology.

Ancient yogis understood the importance of breathing long before heart rate monitors and VO2 max tests existed. They developed Pranayama, a precise science of breath regulation that aims to extend life, optimize vitality, and tap into one's deepest potential. Now, modern science is finally starting to catch up.

Prana means "life force," and yama means "extend or to control." Pranayama is more than merely a series of breathing exercises; it's a holistic practice that unites mind, body, and spirit. It's rooted in the recognition that breath is life. When we breathe deeply, we aren't just drawing in oxygen; we're harmonizing our internal rhythms, soothing our nervous systems, and clearing pathways for emotional and physical healing. As the yogic texts suggest, mastering breath can unlock the doors to heightened awareness, improved health, and longevity.

The slower we breathe, the slower our metabolic rate, which reduces oxidative stress and cellular aging. This is not merely spiritual wisdom, it's rooted in solid physiology. More breaths lead to more oxidative damage, while fewer breaths correlate with increased longevity.

Pranayama reprograms this relationship by reducing the breath rate. This not only slows biological aging but also enhances oxygen efficiency, boosts mitochondrial health, and balances the nervous system, thereby lowering inflammation and stress. Pranayama is a powerful longevity tool disguised as a breathing technique.

Before gyms, supplements, or wearable tech, breath was the first and most potent biohack. Ancient yogis didn't have data, but they had direct experience and understood that how one breathes determines how long and well one lives.

Breath and the Nervous System: The Longevity Switch

Your breath is the key to regulating the autonomic nervous system. Slow, controlled breathing helps shift you from sympathetic dominance, characterized by stress, aging, and inflammation, to parasympathetic mode, which promotes repair, longevity, and deep healing. Fast, shallow breathing is associated with a shorter lifespan due to high cortisol levels, increased oxidative stress, and poor heart rate variability. In contrast, deep, slow breathing contributes to a longer lifespan by lowering inflammation, enhancing oxygen utilization, and improving cellular repair.

Pranayama techniques, such as Nadi Shodhana (alternate nostril breathing) and Bhramari (humming breath), stimulate the vagus nerve. This nerve serves as the parasympathetic brake for stress and aging, and activating it is associated with longevity.

Slow breathing increases heart rate variability (HRV), an essential marker of longevity. Extended exhalations help reduce cortisol levels, lower blood pressure, and improve mitochondrial function. Short intervals of diaphragmatic breathing daily have been shown to boost telomerase activity, the enzyme responsible for repairing and extending telomeres, which are the biological indicator of aging. Pranayama promotes relaxation and rewires the body for a longer, healthier life.

Oxygen Utilization: Why Less is More

We often assume that more oxygen is always better for our bodies, but that's not the case. Both elite endurance athletes and long-living yogis understand a counterintuitive truth: The most efficient breathers take in less oxygen rather than more. Oxygen serves as fuel but is also a highly reactive molecule that can generate oxidative stress.

When you breathe too quickly, shallowly, or through your mouth, you lose carbon dioxide (CO_2), which is essential for effective oxygen absorption. Nasal breathing, on the other hand, increases the production of nitric oxide (NO), which enhances circulation, oxygen delivery, and brain function.

Pranayama techniques, such as Kumbhaka (breath retention), help train the body to use oxygen more efficiently. This practice increases CO_2 tolerance and reduces metabolic wear and tear, which is essential for extending lifespan.

Research shows that higher CO_2 tolerance is associated with lower inflammation, improved brain function, and a reduced risk of chronic disease. Therefore, breathing more slowly optimizes oxygen usage and activates pathways that promote anti-aging.

If you want to slow the aging process, focus on breathing slower.

Pranayama is more than breathwork. It is a comprehensive system designed to enhance the human lifespan, reduce stress, and improve oxygen efficiency. By practicing slow, controlled nasal breathing, occasionally holding your breath (known as Kumbhaka), and balancing your nervous system daily through techniques like Nadi Shodhana, you can activate a biological pathway to longevity that modern medicine is only beginning to comprehend.

As we weave the effects of breath into our daily lives, we recognize that pranayama is not just a series of techniques but a lifestyle choice, an invitation to cultivate greater awareness and health. Every mindful breath allows us to bridge the gap between the mind and body, engaging in a dynamic conversation that fosters balance and resilience.

Your breath is the oldest and most potent primal tool for health and longevity. Want to live longer? Master your breath.

Integrating Body and Mind

Being a neuroradiologist, every brain and spine scan reminds me of our incredible intricacy. The primal design of how these structures relate is even more fascinating. In neuroanatomy class, we learned how specific brain regions are responsible for speech, memory, motor functions, and more. But modern science is discovering that what we call the "mind" is far more complex and fascinating than we initially thought. I often ask my audience a simple question: "Where is your mind located?"

The majority of the crowd will reflexively point to their heads. What a silly question. Our minds are obviously in our heads, right? Everyone knows their brain is the command center of their cognitive and bodily processes. Yet, we see a different story as we look at our primal instincts, the wisdom of Eastern cultures, and ancient yogic traditions. We learn that the concept of mind is more of a collective entity. The mind is localized in the brain and extends throughout every cell in the body. That's right; every cell of our body carries an innate intelligence.

Eastern traditions of India and China have long understood that we think with our brains and whole bodies. Our central nervous system, comprised of our brain and spinal cord, permeates the entire body and influences every aspect of how we perceive and interact with the world. When someone says, "I have a gut feeling," this intuition rises from a more primal locus of intelligence. These deeper forms of intelligence can guide us to a more connected way of living.

Meet Your "Second Brain"

For millennia, Japanese and Indian traditions have focused on the area two inches below the navel as the center of physical and spiritual balance. This center goes by many names, including Hara, Swadhisthana chakra, and Dan Tian.

These ancient traditions have called this neural network the second brain. In martial arts, it is the source of power, stability, and stillness.

Modern science recognizes the significance of this neural network by understanding the "gut-brain axis." Neuroscientists have discovered that the gut hosts a vast network of neurons, almost like a second brain, communicating with our central cognitive centers. This is a high-speed broadband connection where vital information on mood, appetite, and psychological well-being is exchanged.

This gut or enteric nervous system, our "second brain," boasts over 100 million neurons, more than are in our spinal cord. This is a significant finding since what happens here translates into "gut feelings." This ties into the importance of maintaining a healthy gut microbiome, which we discussed earlier. These microbes outnumber human cells and play a crucial role in digesting food, regulating metabolism, and, more importantly, communicating with our brain. The health of our gut microbiome hence plays a vital role in our cognitive, functional, and emotional well-being. This sheds new light on the old advice to "trust your gut!"

The gut-brain axis offers a genuine mind-body connection and a paradigm shift for holistic health. This bidirectional flow highlights the significance of mental health for physical wellness and vice versa. Mental stress can translate into an upset stomach, while poor digestion can lead to nervous thoughts. It's a constant mind-belly dialogue. Researchers continue investigating how targeted therapies, including diet and stress management practices, could optimize this axis for better health outcomes. Let each gut feeling be a reminder of this incredible symbiosis within us.

HeartMath: Tuning into the Rhythm of Your Heart

The HearthMath Institute is a non-profit research and educational organization that explores the impact of heart-brain interactions on health and well-being. Along with the gut-brain exchange, there is a parallel continuous dialogue between the heart and brain. In fact, the heart sends more signals to the brain than vice versa, giving the phrase "follow your heart" a whole new meaning.

This heart-brain dialogue impacts our perception, emotions, and decision-making. Remember those moments when the anticipatory excitement of an event sent your heart racing while you remained perfectly still? Similarly, we all recall those moments when we felt a "heavy heart" reflecting our depressed mental status.

HearthMath Institute researchers pioneered the concept of "heart coherence," a state of synchronization between the heart and mind that leads to improved mental and emotional health. This coherence is not just about feeling good; it transforms the brain's capacity for clarity and enhances intuition and cognitive functioning.

Eastern cultures have always viewed the heart as not just an efficient pump but rather as a source of emotional perception and wisdom. HeartMath researchers find that the heart's rhythms mirror our emotional states. The research reveals how heart coherence, achieved through practices that promote gratitude and compassion, enhance mental clarity and well-being. Imagine your heart and brain dancing in perfect synchrony, where each step enhances emotional control and cognitive performance.

One way of measuring heart coherence is by using heart rate variability (HRV). HRV is a proxy for our stress level and resilience. It captures the rhythm between the beats and represents the variation in time intervals between consecutive heartbeats. While we might think of our heart rate as a consistent rhythm, there is a hidden message between the beats.

Everyone has a unique HRV range. When we operate at the upper limits of our HRV, we are highly adaptable and resilient. At high HRV levels, our autonomic nervous system (ANS) functions at its optimum level, balancing sympathetic ("fight or flight") and parasympathetic ("rest and digest") pathways. Conversely, a low HRV suggests chronic stress, fatigue, or reduced cardiovascular fitness.

Understanding and monitoring HRV can provide greater insight into our health status. If, for example, your HRV drops for several days, it may signal that you're overtraining, undergoing stress, or experiencing a lack of sleep. Modern wearable HRV monitoring devices can offer valuable feedback on our recovery status, stress management, and performance. So, learn to listen to the language of your heart, hidden between the beats. It is there to guide you towards a healthier, more resilient existence.

Wisdom of Head, Heart, and Hara

Our primal intelligence is not isolated in our brain. The gut-brain and heart-brain coherence research we discussed shows that we think with our entire body. We have a perfect trifecta of logic, emotional intelligence, and intuition if we can leverage our intellect, heart sense, and gut instincts. By tapping into our heart intelligence through monitoring HRV and learning to read our gut intuition, we can use modern science to integrate these ancient sources of wisdom. Let's tune into our innate intelligence by aligning our head, heart, and hara to cultivate a life of greater insight, balance, and connection.

The Essence of Yoga: Union

"Yoga" originates from the Sanskrit root "yuj," which means to join or unite. In its purest form, yoga represents the union of the mind and body. It fosters a deep connection within us that synchronizes our physical and mental states. This harmonious union is considered the ultimate formula for well-being.

Yoga encourages us to cultivate awareness of our physical bodies and thoughts in order to bridge the gap that frequently divides them. This unity revitalizes us, enabling us to experience life more fully and consciously and enhances mental clarity and physical health.

Scientific research supports the teachings of Patanjali from centuries ago. Harmonizing the body and mind activates our parasympathetic nervous system and reduces stress hormones like cortisol, restoring balance and promoting health. MRI studies have shown that regular yoga can increase gray matter in brain regions related to stress regulation, empathy, and perspective-taking. Additionally, yoga enhances proprioception, our awareness of the body's position in space, which can help prevent injuries and improve physical performance. This increased body awareness is a direct pathway to enhancing coordination, balance, and mindfulness.

The mind-body connection through yoga is not limited to studio classes. It embodies a way of living in yoga: union. This concept encourages us to integrate this paradigm into our everyday activities, fostering heightened awareness and an intentional way of living.

In essence, yoga is about returning home to ourselves. It invites us back into the present, where genuine connection and healing await.

By calming our inner turbulence, we align with our true nature, living authentically and peacefully. So, the next time you feel the pull of the swirling snowflakes within, remember Patanjali's three words and let them ground you. Set the snow globe down, watch as the flakes settle, and see the world with clear eyes, embracing the perfect simplicity of here and now.

Sleep as a Mind-Body Reset:

Growing up among the Hadzabe, I learned that their sleep quality was crucial for maintaining physical and mental health. Over the years, I've observed how modern society has disrupted our primal sleep patterns and rhythms through technological advancements and lifestyle changes.

Disruption of Circadian Rhythms

Emerging research highlights sleep as an essential component of optimal health, on par with nutrition and exercise. Quality sleep plays a vital role in our biological functions and emotional well-being. Our bodies operate on circadian rhythms that align with the Earth's natural light-dark cycle. Unfortunately, modern advancements often disrupt these rhythms, leading to significant health consequences.

As a radiologist, I constantly stare at a screen during work hours, as do many professionals today. Interestingly, artificial lighting, combined with this constant exposure to screens, particularly in the evenings, impairs our ability to produce melatonin, the hormone responsible for initiating restorative sleep. Exposure to blue light at night from fluorescent bulbs and LED screens signals our brains that it is still daytime, which suppresses melatonin production. This delay in melatonin release can hinder our ability to fall asleep and reduce sleep quality. Consequently, our sleep becomes fragmented, weakening the mind-body connection. Quality sleep is crucial for memory consolidation, emotional regulation, and physical recovery.

Chronic Sleep Deprivation

Compared to life in the African savanna, our modern lifestyle prioritizes productivity over restful sleep. The recommended seven to nine hours of sleep feels like a distant fantasy for most people. However, scientific evidence indicates insufficient sleep is associated with a higher mortality risk. Operating on less than six hours of sleep consistently has been linked to numerous health risks, including an increased likelihood of heart disease. There is currently an epidemic of sleep deprivation that stresses the body and reduces its ability to communicate effectively with the mind, creating a divide in the mind-body connection. Sleep is sacrificed for late-night work, mindless social media scrolling, and streaming entertainment.

Chronic lack of sleep is a modern-age issue with many consequences. Our early ancestors had no choice but to hit the sack when the sun went down. Our modern sleep-robbing conveniences take a toll on our mental faculties, dulling cognitive function, stifling creativity, and impairing decision-making abilities. Our immune defenses suffer, leaving us susceptible to illness as inflammation quietly simmers beneath the surface. Impaired sleep disrupts our metabolic control and hormonal balance, leading to weight gain and metabolic disorders.

Rediscovering Natural Rhythms

Sleep is not merely a period of rest, but a symphony composed of distinct cycles, each playing a crucial role in maintaining harmony within our minds and bodies. Living closely with nature, the Hadzabe experience optimal sleep cycles, guided by the sun's rise and setting rather than by digital clocks. Because they do not experience the cacophony of modern stressors, their sleep follows nature's rhythm, becoming full, restorative, and harmonious. This natural confluence supports their vitality, showcasing the innate wisdom of aligning with Earth's cycles.

But why is sleep so important for our brain's well-being? Beyond feeling rested, sleep serves as a cognitive housekeeper. During deep sleep, particularly in the slow-wave stage, the brain detoxifies, clearing out metabolic waste and "brain debris" like beta-amyloid, which, if allowed to accumulate, is associated with conditions like Alzheimer's disease.

Simultaneously, sleep is crucial for memory consolidation. During this nightly journey, the brain decides what to hold onto and what to discard. Imagine Marie Kondo tidying up your synaptic connections. Solidifying important information and discarding the nonsense helps us operate more efficiently.

The Stages of Sleep:

1. **Stage 1 (Light Sleep):** This stage transitions us from wakefulness to sleep. Our muscles relax, and our breathing slows, signaling the body to prepare for deeper stages.

2. **Stage 2 (Deeper Light):** The heart rate and temperature drop at this stage.

3. **Stage 3 (Slow-Wave Sleep):** Often referred to as deep sleep, this stage is the mainstay of recuperation and rejuvenation. During this stage, the body repairs tissues, builds bone and muscle, and strengthens the immune system.

4. **REM Sleep (Rapid Eye Movement):** REM sleep is where dreams flourish. During this phase, the brain sorts through emotions and consolidates memories. It's a critical period for mental and emotional processing, where the mind pieces things together and finds creative solutions.

Contrast this natural order with the fragmented sleep of modern life's 24/7 demands. Chronic stress leads to elevated cortisol levels, which disrupt these harmonious sleep stages. Fragmented sleep interferes with critical slow-wave and REM sleep, denying us the full quality of rest we need. As sleep cycles become dysfunctional, our ability to restore and regenerate diminishes, resulting in fatigue, heightened anxiety, and diminished resilience.

Why We Can't Sleep Like Our Ancestors

You can track your macros, biohack your way through cold plunges, and drink all the green smoothies you want, but if your sleep is broken, so are you. Yet, here we are, a society running on caffeine, cortisol, and sleep debt, treating rest like an optional luxury rather than a biological necessity. The primal truth? **We were designed to sleep deeply, effortlessly, and in sync with the rhythms of nature.** But somewhere between artificial lights, late-night Netflix binges, and the 24/7 hustle, we forgot how.

Our ancestors didn't need melatonin gummies or white noise machines. They woke with the sun, moved all day, and when darkness fell, their bodies naturally slipped into deep, restorative sleep. Their circadian rhythms were locked into nature's cycles, with no blue light, no alarm clocks, no endless doom-scrolling. But today? We live in an environment our biology doesn't recognize.

Artificial Light Confusion:

Every morning, sunlight floods our eyes, signaling our brain's internal clock to elevate cortisol levels, which helps us wake up and stay alert. At the same time, it suppresses melatonin, preventing sleep, and ignites our metabolism, indicating it's time to move and eat. At night, this process reverses: cortisol levels drop, indicating it's time to repair and recover, melatonin levels rise, preparing us for sleep, and our core body temperature decreases, setting the stage for deep sleep.

However, we have replaced natural sunlight with screens and moonlight with LED bulbs. The blue light emitted by phones and TVs tricks our brains into thinking it is still daytime, suppressing melatonin production and delaying our ability to sleep at night. This leaves our primal bodies caught in a digital world.

Lack of Movement = Poor Sleep:

Our ancestors walked 8 to 10 miles a day, engaging in activities like hunting, gathering, climbing, squatting, lifting, and running. They earned their sleep through physical movement. In contrast, modern humans often sit for over 12 hours a day and then wonder why they struggle to sleep.

When we exercise, our bodies use energy and break down ATP (adenosine triphosphate), releasing adenosine as a byproduct. Adenosine binds to receptors in the brain, signaling the need for sleep. Engaging in physical activity during the day enhances slow-wave sleep, a crucial period during which our bodies repair and regenerate.

Overstimulated Brains:

Our ancestors dealt with occasional acute, short-term stress from predators and hunger. In contrast, we experience chronic stress from emails, deadlines, and traffic. As a result, cortisol levels remain high while melatonin levels are low. Brains overstimulated by social media, news, and digital distractions hijack our nervous systems, making it impossible to achieve deep sleep.

Inconsistent Sleep Schedules:

We go to bed and wake up at random times, disrupting the master clock that regulates our sleep-wake cycles. Your body is a rhythm machine. Sleeping at random times is like switching time zones daily, so your circadian rhythm never stabilizes.

Caffeine and Stimulants:

To combat the fatigue caused by our busy lives, we often rely on caffeine and stimulants as quick fixes. A morning cup can necessitate an afternoon boost, creating a cycle of dependency. While these substances may help us feel temporarily alert, their effects can linger, disrupting our natural sleep patterns. Caffeine, in particular, negatively impacts total sleep duration, especially by interfering with deep and restorative sleep. It binds to the adenosine receptors discussed earlier, reducing deep sleep signals. Additionally, residual caffeine in our system increases neuronal activity at night, making us more alert and stimulated.

Deep sleep isn't a luxury, it's a biological necessity. It governs memory,

metabolism, immunity, and longevity. But the modern world has built an anti-sleep environment, and we are suffering for it. The solution? Rewild your sleep. Follow the primal laws of light, movement, and timing, and watch your energy, focus, and health transform.

Want to sleep like an optimized human? Live like one.

Mind-Body Unity: From Chaos to Clarity

The mind is a relentless time traveler. It drags us into the wreckage of the past, sifting through regrets, replaying old failures, rewriting what-ifs. Or it hurls us into the uncertain future, where anxieties multiply like fractals, expanding into fears that may never materialize. Meanwhile, life—the real, breathing, pulsing moment—slips by unnoticed.

The true purpose of mastering the mind-body connection is not just better health, lower cortisol, or a more efficient nervous system. Those are byproducts. The real goal is clarity, a mind that is sharp, present, and fully engaged with life as it is, not as the mind distorts it.

Science confirms what ancient wisdom has long known:

When the mind and body are in sync, we see reality more clearly.

The HeartMath Institute shows us that when our heart rhythms are coherent, synchronized with deep, calm emotions, we process information better, make wiser decisions, and move through life with greater ease. The gut-brain axis reminds us that what we eat and how we nourish our microbiome influences our emotions, instincts, and resilience. Sleep resets our brain, clearing out mental fog and recalibrating perception. Conscious breathing is our most immediate tool, every inhale and exhale anchoring us to the now.

Every day, I review CT scans and radiographs, real-time snapshots of a person's health. They strip away all illusions. You may tell yourself that you're "getting back in shape soon," but the scan tells me how your organs are functioning right now. You may have good intentions about improving your diet, but your arteries, your liver, and your bones don't care about intentions. They reflect your present reality. There is no past in a radiograph, no hopeful future, only this moment. This is clarity.

Once we embrace clarity, we can chart a more effective course. Just as a CT scan provides a clear assessment of internal health, mindful awareness gives us a truthful image of our mental and emotional state. If we constantly experience stress, resentment, or distraction, our nervous system reflects that, whether we acknowledge it or not. But we can make meaningful changes once we see things as they are.

This is why conscious breathing is so powerful. Every breath exists only in the present. You cannot inhale for yesterday or exhale for tomorrow. Each breath is a direct encounter with reality. **The more we practice being present with the breath, the more we train ourselves to stay grounded in the now.**

When we align our body and mind, clarity is the natural result. We see people as they are, not as projections of our past wounds. We engage with life fully instead of sleepwalking through it. We stop chasing happiness as some future destination and recognize it in the space between this inhale and the next.

The shift from chaos to clarity isn't a single event, it's a practice. It's in the way we breathe, the way we move, the way we wake up and decide, over and over again, to be here. Now. Because this moment is the only one that's real.

Agitation to Attention to Awareness: The Journey from Mind to No-Mind

In today's world, distraction is the default state of the mind. We are bombarded by notifications, emails, and dopamine-triggering digital breadcrumbs, all conditioning our brains to exist in perpetual fragmentation. Multitasking, once touted as a skill of the elite, is a myth. Neuroscience confirms that when we attempt to split our attention, we don't do two things at once, we just do two things poorly. The prefrontal cortex, responsible for higher cognition, doesn't truly multitask; it rapidly switches between tasks, like a glitching machine, leading to cognitive overload and decreased performance. It's no wonder so many people live in a state of low-grade agitation, never fully immersed, never fully present.

This agitation isn't just digital, it is emotional. Almost all negative emotions are temporal distortions. Regret, resentment, and anger anchor us to the past, while anxiety, fear, and worry catapult us into the future. Very rarely do we engage with the only moment that actually exists, the present.

Consider how we work and interact: glancing at texts in meetings, checking our phones mid-conversation, and eating while scrolling. This fractured attention keeps us from experiencing the world as it is. The solution isn't adding more to our cognitive plate but subtracting the noise, refining our ability to hold attention and transition into deep awareness.

The Science of Deep Work

In his seminal work, Deep Work, Cal Newport discusses how true productivity and mastery emerge only when we enter a state of intense, uninterrupted focus. Neuroscience backs this. The myelination of neural pathways, the process that strengthens and accelerates brain function, occurs most effectively in deep work states. When we single-task, our neurons fire in coherent patterns, reinforcing efficiency. The opposite happens in distraction: Fragmented inputs prevent the brain from building efficient pathways, leaving us mentally scattered and exhausted.

Athletes, musicians, and master craftspeople understand this intuitively. My son, a pianist, doesn't simply "practice." He repeats a passage hundreds of times until his fingers move with their own mind. Flow emerges when attention becomes so stabilized that action and awareness merge. There is no more "trying," just doing. The woodworkers in my lineage knew this too. The first strokes with a chisel are deliberate and thoughtful. But over time, the hands know before the mind does. The best carvers don't think about shaving away wood; they feel the grain and move harmoniously. The mind quiets. Only awareness remains.

Sat Chit Anand: From Attention to Awareness

In my Indian heritage, there is the term Sat Chit Anand. Roughly translated, it means truth-consciousness-bliss, or being fully awake to the present moment's joy. Many in my family greet each other with this phrase, a reminder of what matters. It is a map of the journey we must take:

1. **Agitation to Attention**—The first step is to break free from distraction and bring awareness to something singular: the breath, the flicker of a flame, a mantra. Thoughts still arise in this stage, but we tether ourselves to the present despite them. The mind resists, but repetition rewires it.

2. **Attention to Awareness**—As attention stabilizes over time, awareness deepens. This is where deep work, meditation, and peak performance overlap. The distractions fade, and the present moment expands. Here, a pianist plays not with effort but instinct; a runner feels not the exertion, but the rhythm; and a meditator is no longer "meditating" but simply existing.

3. **Awareness to No-Mind**—The final paradox is that the mind must dissolve to be truly aware. Here, you enter flow, a state where you are fully alive. The Hadzabe effortlessly embodied this state. When tracking an animal, they were fully immersed, no thoughts of past failures, no anxiety about future outcomes, only raw presence. In those moments, they became the hunt, the landscape, the very breath in their lungs.

Essentially, the mind must focus enough to dissolve itself and ultimately experience life. Only by relinquishing the ego, by surrendering the illusion of separation, does one achieve true awareness and transcendence. In the same way, meditation and the mind-body connection lead us to a place where the mind is no longer an obstacle but a gateway to pure presence and deep living.

We must arrive at this space, the space beyond thought and worry. **The mind and body are connected so well that they can step aside, allowing life to**

unfold in its most vivid, unfiltered form. This is where we live, not in the past or the future but in the pulsing immediacy of now.

Primal Practices:

Stillness isn't just the absence of noise; it's the ability to remain centered, grounded, and fully present, no matter what's happening around you. In a world designed to pull you into constant stimulation, developing stillness is a radical act of self-mastery. It's also a biological necessity, linked to lower cortisol, increased neuroplasticity, and longevity.

Here are seven key daily approaches to cultivating stillness, drawn from both primal wisdom and modern neuroscience.

1. Morning Silence (No External Inputs for the First 30 Minutes)

The way you start your day sets the foundation for your brain's operating system. If you wake up and immediately check your phone, emails, or the news, your nervous system gets overwhelmed by external demands before you even get out of bed.

In the first 30 minutes of your day, try to avoid your phone, notifications, and news. Instead, drink water, move slowly, and breathe deeply. You can read, reflect, or simply sit in stillness. This practice helps reset your dopamine sensitivity, preventing compulsive phone checking and reducing the cortisol surge caused by digital overstimulation. It also creates a mental space before the outside world begins to intrude.

2. The 4-Second Rule (Pausing Before Reacting)

Most of us tend to react rather than respond. We quickly send emails, jump into conversations, and make decisions without pausing between the stimulus and our response. This can lead to mental clutter and increased stress. Before you reply, make a decision, or engage in conflict, take a moment to pause for four seconds. Inhale . . . Hold . . . Exhale . . . then respond. This practice activates the prefrontal cortex, promoting higher reasoning and reducing reactivity. It helps you gain control over emotional impulses and cultivates mental clarity in your daily life.

3. Single-Tasking (Eliminate Mental Fragmentation)

Multitasking destroys focus and inner peace. It increases cortisol levels because the brain perceives multitasking as a threat. This behavior reduces your ability to engage in deep work, leaving you feeling mentally scattered.

To improve focus, try these strategies: tackle one task at a time, avoid using your phone while working, refrain from scrolling through social media while eating, and don't check emails during conversations.

Utilize time blocks, such as dedicating **90 minutes to deep work followed by a 30-minute break.** Silence notifications to train your brain to concentrate better.

Adopting these practices can strengthen one's attentional control, help one enter a flow state more easily, and reduce mental fatigue. This ultimately fosters a deep sense of stillness, even while working.

4. Breathwork: Longevity Protocol

Daily Longevity Breath (6:6:6:6 Box Breathing): Inhale for 6 seconds, hold, exhale, and hold, all for 6 seconds each. Repeat for 5-10 minutes daily to slow aging, increase CO_2 tolerance, and enhance mitochondrial function.

Nadi Shodhana (Alternate Nostril Breathing): Engage in alternate nostril breathing for 5 minutes to balance the nervous system, lower cortisol, and increase heart rate variability (HRV).

Kumbhaka (Breath Retention): Practice inhaling deeply, holding until slight discomfort, and exhaling fully. Repeat circles to boost oxygen efficiency, nitric oxide, and lung function.

Your breath is the remote control for your nervous system. Most people breathe too fast and shallow, keeping their minds restless.

5. Digital Detox Windows (Scheduled Tech-Free Time)

Stillness cannot exist in a world filled with constant notifications. Your brain needs mental white space to process, reflect, and restore clarity. Aim for two hours per day without screens; that's less than 10% of your 24-hour day. Spend this time outside, take a walk, or engage in something completely non-digital. As a bonus, try to have one full tech-free day each week (a Digital Sabbath). This practice can reset your dopamine sensitivity, reduce compulsive phone checking, improve your attention span, and enhance your ability to be present. It also helps you regain a sense of time and depth in life.

6. Mindfulness and the Art of Breathing: Anapanasati Yoga

Even 5-10 minutes of conscious breathing can rewire your brain for calmness, focus, and clarity. Approach this practice without expectations and simply observe your thoughts as if they are passing clouds. Mindful breathing thickens the prefrontal cortex, which helps reduce impulsivity and anxiety. It also increases gray matter density, contributing to brain longevity. Finally, it trains the mind to find stillness anywhere, at any time.

Anapanasati Yoga offers a transformative journey toward inner peace and awareness. Enjoy each breath as you anchor yourself in the present moment, embracing the many layers of mindfulness that this ancient practice provides.

Morning Respite:

Start your day with 5-10 minutes of mindful breathing. Find a quiet, comfortable spot, perhaps a serene corner or by a window. Focus on your natural breath and observe the sensation of air entering and leaving your nostrils. This practice sets a calm and centered tone for the day.

Midday Check-In:

In the midst of your daily hustle, take a few moments to reconnect with your breath. Close your eyes and take slow, deep breaths, paying attention to the rise and fall of your chest. This brief pause offers a mental reset, enhancing your focus and presence for the afternoon ahead.

Walking Meditation:

Combine Anapanasati with movement during a leisurely walk. Synchronize your breathing with your steps: inhale for three steps, pause, then exhale for three. Walking in nature can enhance this experience, transforming a simple stroll into a meditative practice that unites body and mind.

Evening Unwind:

Dedicate some time in the evening to a more extended Anapanasati session, aiming for 10 to 20 minutes. Focus on the depth of your breath and the transitions between inhales and exhales. This practice promotes relaxation, helping you release the day's stressors and prepare for restful sleep.

7. The Primal Sleep Reset (Power Down the Mind)

Morning Sunlight: Get outside within 30 minutes of waking up to help anchor your circadian clock. Avoid wearing sunglasses or having windows block the sun's natural light.

Ditch Blue Light at Night: After sunset, choose red lights, candles, or dim, warm lighting instead of screens. Try to avoid screens for 90 minutes before bedtime to prepare your body for rest.

Move Like a Hunter-Gatherer: Incorporate natural movements into your daily routine (walking, lifting, stretching, squatting, and playing). Make movement an essential part of your life.

Cool Your Core Body Temperature: Sleep in a cool room (65–67°F). Consider taking a cold shower or soaking your feet before bed to initiate sleep.

Consistent Sleep-Wake Times: To stabilize your rhythm, maintain regular sleep and wake times. Aim to go to bed and wake up within the same 30-minute window each day, even on weekends.

Final Thought: Stillness through the mind-body connection is a skill, not a coincidence. In a world that thrives on distraction and busyness, you cultivate stillness intentionally.

Choose one or two of these practices to start today. Over time, you may notice increased mental clarity, reduced stress and reactivity, and a deeper sense of presence. True stillness isn't about escaping the world but mastering your inner world so that external chaos no longer controls you.

Be still to be purposeful, as we discover next.

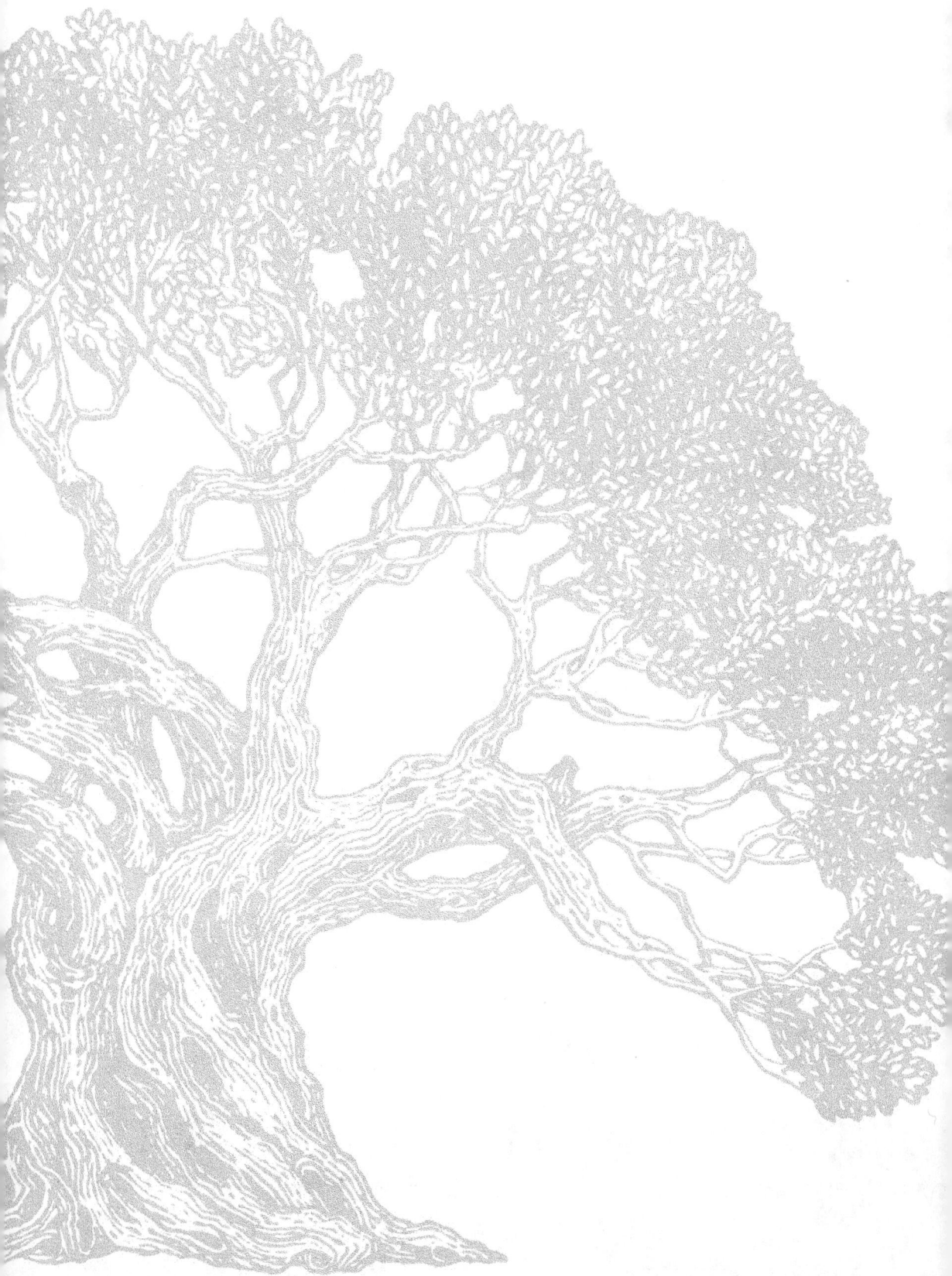

5

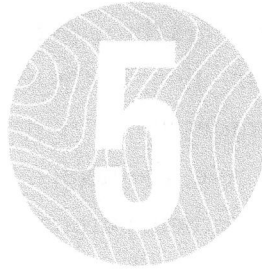

THE SEED OF PURPOSE: FINDING YOUR IKIGAI

"Your purpose in life is to find your purpose and give your whole heart and soul to it."
– Buddha.

Primal Purpose: Ancient Blueprint for Fulfillment

In the heart of the African wilderness, among the vibrant tapestry of tribal cultures, I witnessed a simplicity and clarity that left an indelible mark. Each individual knew their role, and harmony sang through the tribe, each person leveraging their unique strengths towards a collective goal. No one appeared confused about their purpose; like instruments in an orchestra, they played their parts in flawless symphony.

In Indian tradition, it is believed that each person is born with a unique constitution; some are highly intellectual, others physically adept, many emotionally sensitive, and a few are driven by introspection. This inclination is not a modern conception but a timeless reverberation felt deep within our biology.

Our ancestral narratives are abundant with purpose, an understanding so vital that it guided our ancestors through the challenges of the unknown. The purpose was more than ambition; it was a necessary navigation tool in a world where forming communities and overcoming obstacles required cooperation and clear roles. Each role, the healer, the hunter, the gatherer, was indispensable to the tribe, and their purposes were intimately interwoven with survival.

Biologically, our brains are finely tuned to align with purposeful actions. Neuroscience tells us that a sense of purpose enhances neurochemicals like dopamine, a natural high that fosters resilience and long-term satisfaction. When early humans set out on a hunt or gathered resources, their purposeful work was mentally and physically rewarding, a feedback loop that ensured survival and well-being.

Purpose is intertwined with our primal urge for belonging and social connection. In tribal societies, roles were clearly defined, and each contribution held significance. This ensured physical survival and fortified mental health, fulfilling the deep-seated need to contribute and belong.

However, modern society often dilutes this instinct. The cacophony of distractions and superficial pursuits muddles our intrinsic purposes, leaving many in a sea of uncertainty. The result? A disconnection from the evolutionary blueprint crafted to support our thriving.

Identifying a clear purpose can lend a profound sense of direction. By tapping into our ancient roots, individuals may find greater fulfillment and align their modern lives with a path that supports and celebrates their unique gifts.

As we embark on the journey to find your ikigai, remember that purpose is not about discovering a single grand life mission but about engaging with what resonates deeply within you. Let us embrace the roles we were born to play, leveraging them to build thriving communities and foster a life of both personal and collective significance.

The Dilemma: Modern Man's Quest for Meaning

Ancient societies had a knack for identifying specific roles based on traditions and individual strengths. Each tribe member understood how their talents served the greater good; an effortless sense of belonging attached to the heartbeat of their community. Fast-forward to today's hyper-competitive landscape, and you will find a sea of individuals adrift, unsure of how they fit into the vast world around them.

In our modern milieu, the interdependence and clarity once guiding our ancestors seem disrupted. Instead, many seek validation from the superficial standards set by social media, where the comparison game runs rampant. Who has not felt the pressure to conform to someone else's scripted version of success, to let job titles define purpose rather than authentic calling?

Journey to Meaning

Viktor Frankl was no ordinary psychiatrist; he was a beacon of resilience wrapped in the pages of history. Born in Vienna in 1905, Frankl's fascination with the human mind ran deep from an early age. However, his harrowing experiences during World War II shaped his philosophy and led him to write the pivotal book *Man's Search for Meaning,* one of my life-changing reads.

As the Nazi regime increased its control over Europe, Viktor Frankl, a Jewish psychiatrist, faced unimaginable circumstances. Stripped of his career, he was detained in Auschwitz and later transferred to other concentration camps. In this horrific environment, he witnessed the remarkable strength of the human spirit when confronted with despair.

Frankl noticed that those who managed to cling to hope, be it a memory of a loved one, a goal to achieve, or even a semblance of purpose, were far more likely to survive than those who succumbed to despair. He called this phenomenon the "will to meaning."

Frankl formulated his groundbreaking theories in the depths of suffering, which gave birth to the concept of "existential emptiness." This term refers to a void left gaping as traditional anchors of purpose erode, leaving many floundering in the vastness of choice. The condition is exacerbated by the modern world's complexities and societal pressures, where meaning is not handed down by elders but must be excavated from within.

Frankl's life story reminds us that while challenges are inevitable, the quest for meaning is like a lifeline in rough seas. His insights resonate through time, teaching us that even in our darkest moments, pursuing purpose can light our way and help us forge connections that sustain life. Frankl's journey illustrates that finding meaning can transform our struggles into stepping-stones, guiding us toward a more fulfilling existence.

What Do We Live For?

Reflecting on our ancestral lives, we see that purpose was intrinsically tied to survival and tribe welfare. In contrast, modern conveniences have obliterated the struggle to survive, leaving many questioning what they live for, if not survival.

They say we are born twice: once on our birthdate and again when we discover our true reason for being. In an era of ease and comfort, the challenge is not merely survival but uncovering and embracing what fuels our passion and sense of purpose. As we transition into this journey of self-discovery, it is time to peel back the layers obscuring true calling and shine a light on our authentic purpose, a gem unshackled from external validation and rooted instead in personal truth.

The Tough Journey of Finding Purpose

Growing up, it felt like I was on an endless treasure hunt, but no one had told me what I was searching for. My father was an engineer, and I thought I would have inherited some mysterious knack for mechanics alongside my DNA. My grades would make any parent beam proud, landing me a spot in a top honors engineering program. However, my first real engineering class (Vector Dynamics, to be exact) was a ruthless wake-up call. The formulas did not jive with me; they put me to sleep.

Realizing I was not cut out for solving equations resembling ancient hieroglyphs, I quit the honors program. I switched gears, opting for a biology major. However, biology had its concrete paths: a lab rat or a doctor. I chose the latter, carving out a space for myself in medicine.

Even within the world of healthcare, I still felt adrift, like a lone buoy bobbing in the sea of diagnostic radiology. Each evening on-call shift seemed like an endless loop of shades and shadows with no definitive end. Fulfillment eluded me until I redirected my focus to teaching and mentoring.

That is when it clicked. My forte is translating complex medical concepts into digestible, practical information for medical students and residents. I envision helping the next generation of doctors weave these narratives into their expanding medical knowledge base. Among the shades of gray, I unearthed a calling, a thread connecting complexity with clarity.

I discovered this passion was not limited to clinical practice; it spilled into health speaking. My knack for distilling the latest medical research into practical wisdom could empower everyday living. This journey, this blend of teaching and guiding, eventually led me to express my findings as an author, building a bridge between clinical practice, our primal intelligence, and the daily dance of life.

The road to finding purpose is undeniably tough, and everyone takes a different path. There is no universal "right" or "wrong" way; it is just your way. The anchor came through the Japanese tradition of ikigai, a convergence of what I love, what I am good at, what the world needs, and what I can be paid for. This philosophy nurtured my search for purpose, turning a meandering quest into a meaningful voyage.

We all have our unique journeys. Mine led to a place where purpose and passion intersect, offering both a challenge and a reward, a perpetual sense of discovery and fulfillment.

Life of Purpose: Finding Your Ikigai

Ikigai is a Japanese concept that embodies the intersection of one's passions, talents, values, and contributions to the world. It provides a sense of purpose and reason for being. Originating from the Japanese words "ki" (life) and "gai" (worth or value), ikigai roughly translates to "a reason for living."

Historically, ikigai has roots in Japanese culture and philosophy, particularly in Okinawa, a region known for its high concentration of centenarians. Okinawans often attribute their longevity and happiness to having a strong sense of purpose, or ikigai, which guides their daily activities and interactions. In Okinawan culture, ikigai is less about individual achievement and more about contributing to one's family and community, living in alignment with nature, and nurturing social relationships.

In its modern interpretation, ikigai is often represented as the overlap of four elements:

1. **What you love** – your passions and interests.

2. **What you are good at** – your skills and strengths.

3. **What the world needs** – your potential to contribute meaningfully.

4. **What you can be paid for** – an element of practicality and financial sustainability.

When these elements align, they reveal a fulfilling path that sustains motivation and well-being. While the Western interpretation sometimes emphasizes professional fulfillment, ikigai in Japan remains more personal and introspective. It focuses on enjoying small pleasures, engaging in meaningful work, and contributing to others' happiness.

By defining and nurturing ikigai, people can connect more deeply with their sense of purpose and life's intrinsic meaning. This concept aligns closely with the primal desire to live purposefully.

The Science of Flow and the Path to Purpose

A rare yet unmistakable feeling occurs when you become so deeply immersed in an activity that time seems to dissolve, your sense of self fades away, and effort transforms into pure ease. This state is known as "flow," and it may be one of the most overlooked pathways to finding purpose in modern life. Neuroscientists use functional MRI scans to observe how the brain operates during these moments. Regions associated with self-criticism quiet down, while networks linked to creativity and deep focus become highly active. Though neuroscientists refer to this phenomenon as transient hypofrontality, it can simply be described as the art of being fully alive.

Flow is a concept popularized by psychologist Mihaly Csikszentmihalyi, who described it as a mental state where individuals are entirely immersed in an activity, often with a loss of time and the outside world. It is not merely about doing something you enjoy; it is about doing something that challenges you just enough to keep you engaged without overwhelming you. Scientific studies reveal that during flow, our brains release a mix of neurochemicals such as dopamine and endorphins, enhancing focus and joy.

During my time with the Hadzabe, I noticed something striking. Whether tracking an animal, making fire, or crafting a bow, they weren't merely *doing* these activities, they were *becoming* them. There was no overthinking, no hesitation, just an instinctual merging with the task. This is the primal origin of flow. Our ancestors didn't need meditation retreats to experience presence; survival was a complete engagement.

Today, functional MRI scans of elite athletes, musicians, and artists reveal a common neurological pattern when they are in flow: The prefrontal cortex, the part of the brain responsible for self-doubt and overanalysis, quietly steps aside, allowing deeper, instinct-driven networks to take control. It's as if the conscious mind hands the reins to something far older and wiser.

Finding Flow, Finding Purpose

My wife found this truth early. Since the age of three, give her a drawing pen and paper, and the world around her would vanish. She didn't need to be told to practice; she *lived* in the act of creation. Fortunately, her parents recognized this and nurtured her passion. Today, art is not just her career, it is her oxygen.

Most people, however, aren't as lucky. They drift through life, disconnected from the activities that ignite their deepest focus. The key to finding purpose isn't about sitting down and pondering *what I should do with my life*. But instead, it is saying, "I would like to observe *where time disappears for me*." Purpose is revealed through flow. When you find that activity where effort becomes effortless, you are knocking on the door of your life's work.

In grappling with my own life's direction, I discovered just how powerful finding this flow could be. Through trial and error, I identified the activities that resonated most with me: speaking, teaching, and mentoring. Standing before an eager audience or breaking down complex concepts into relatable narratives felt less like work and more like a labor of love. I felt truly alive in these moments, whether on stage or in a one-on-one session. Untethered by time, comfortably curious, and deeply connected to the material and the people around me, I was in flow.

Reflecting on these experiences offered illuminating insights. The episodes where I effortlessly reached flow provided clues about where my passion lay, not in the confines of a lab or the rigid structures of vector dynamics, but in the dynamic interplay of ideas and human connections. It taught me that what brings us to this meditative space often points towards our true passions, and therein lies our purpose.

How to Discover Your Life-Affirming Flow and Purpose

1. Identify Peak Moments of Engagement

- When do you lose track of time? What activity leaves you feeling energized rather than drained? Look for patterns in your past. What did you love doing as a child before the world told you what was "practical"?

2. Follow Curiosity, Not Just Passion

- Passion is often the byproduct of repeated immersion, not the starting point. If you don't know what drives you, follow your curiosity and expose yourself to different experiences.

3. Minimize Distraction, Maximize Deep Work

- Flow requires immersion. In a world of constant pings and notifications, you must create spaces of uninterrupted focus. The more deeply you engage, the closer you will be to uncovering what truly moves you.

4. Pay Attention to Physical & Emotional Signals

- Flow isn't just in the mind; it's in the body. Notice when you feel an effortless rhythm, where your energy is high, and your mind is clear. Purpose doesn't feel like pushing a boulder uphill; it feels like moving with the current.

5. Cultivate Mastery

- Purpose and flow thrive at the intersection of challenge and skill. If an activity is too easy, you get bored. Too hard, you get frustrated. The goal is to engage in something challenging enough to push you, but within reach enough to improve.

The deepest levels of flow transcend thinking altogether. It's no longer effort, it's instinct. The same is true for any master: the woodworker shaping a perfect joint, the surgeon performing with precision, the Hadzabe tracker reading the land as if it were his own body.

To be in flow is to be in harmony with your nature, and when you align with that, purpose is not something you seek, it's something that reveals itself.

We were not designed to exist in distraction and fragmented attention. Our ancestors didn't wake up to scroll through their worries; they woke up to engage with life. If you want to find purpose, step away from the noise. **Find what makes you disappear because, in that disappearance, you will find your true self.** The journey to purpose is the journey to flow, and when you find flow, you find the life you were meant to live.

The Science of Purpose—A Biological Imperative

In the grand architecture of human biology, purpose is not an abstract luxury but a deeply embedded survival mechanism. It is a primal drive encoded in our nervous system, influencing everything from cellular repair to cognitive resilience. Modern neuroscience and longevity research are only now beginning to catch up with what ancient wisdom traditions have always known:

A clear sense of purpose has the power to shape not just our mindset but our very physiology.

Why Purposeful People Live Longer

Take a page from *The Blue Zones*, a book that explores the unique areas around the globe where people live significantly longer and healthier lives. Researchers have found that longevity is not just about environmental factors or genetics; it is deeply intertwined with an individual's sense of purpose. Studies show that people who define their lives with purpose live longer and often enjoy lower incidences of chronic diseases, including Alzheimer's.

Studies find that a stronger purpose in life is associated with decreased all-cause mortality. This is not simply a coincidence; it is a testament to the physiological effects of purpose on our bodies. When you know your "why," you foster a foundation of resilience that mitigates stress, enhances mental health, and positively influences various aspects of well-being.

One of the most compelling scientific cases for the power of purpose comes from Japan, particularly the Okinawan centenarians we discussed, who embody the concept of *ikigai*, a reason for being. Studies have shown that individuals who clearly define their ikigai tend to live longer, healthier lives. The Ohsaki Study, published in 2008, followed over 40,000 Japanese adults and found that those with a strong sense of purpose had significantly lower mortality rates, even when controlling for lifestyle factors like diet and exercise.

Purpose reduces chronic stress, regulates immune function, and promotes psychological resilience. It acts as a biological stabilizer, buffering against the wear and tear of daily life and ultimately extending healthspan.

Neurobiology of Purpose—How Meaning Rewires the Brain

Neuroscience suggests that having a strong sense of meaning doesn't just make life more fulfilling, it fundamentally rewires the brain, optimizing it for focus, resilience, and longevity.

Dopamine, the brain's primary neurotransmitter for motivation and reward, is intimately tied to purposeful action. When we engage in work that aligns with our intrinsic values, whether it's a surgeon saving lives, a woodworker sculpting a masterpiece, or a Hadzabe hunter tracking game, dopamine pathways in the brain light up like a well-worn trail. These pathways reinforce behaviors that lead to deep engagement, making purpose-driven activities neurologically rewarding.

Serotonin, often dubbed the "happiness neurotransmitter," plays a complementary role. Unlike dopamine, which spikes in anticipation of rewards, serotonin fosters a deep, sustained sense of contentment. Studies have shown that people who engage in meaningful work have naturally higher serotonin levels, leading to reduced stress, increased well-being, and greater emotional resilience. This is why doing something that matters, whether treating patients, crafting art, or building a legacy, creates a self-sustaining cycle of purpose and fulfillment.

Neuroimaging has revealed that people with a strong sense of purpose have heightened activity in the prefrontal cortex, the brain's command center for focus, decision-making, and emotional regulation. This makes sense: When we operate with a clear mission, our brain shifts from scattered, reactive thinking to structured, intentional processing. Purpose strengthens executive function, reducing impulsivity and increasing our ability to tackle complex challenges with clarity and precision.

Neuroscience points to differences in brain health between those who live meaningful, purpose-driven lives and those who drift without clear direction.

Studies find that older adults with a high sense of purpose in life exhibit better cognitive function despite the burden of Alzheimer's disease, which manifests as amyloid deposition and nerve tangles. These studies suggest that purpose is an emotional state and a neurological framework for resilience.

The default mode network (DMN) is the brain's background processing system, responsible for mind-wandering, self-referential thoughts, and unfortunately, excessive rumination. When overactive, the DMN fuels negative self-talk, anxiety, and indecision, pulling us into cycles of doubt and distraction. However, studies show that engaging in deeply meaningful activities suppresses the DMN and enhances present-moment awareness.

Purpose as Medicine

Purpose is not just a mindset but a hormonal switch that can recalibrate our entire nervous system. Chronic stress and lack of direction elevate cortisol, the primary stress hormone, leading to inflammation, insulin resistance, and accelerated aging. Purpose, however, activates the parasympathetic nervous system by lowering heart rate, reducing inflammation, and promoting metabolic efficiency.

Chronic inflammation is a crucial contributor to cardiovascular issues. Stress, a significant driver of inflammation, tends to diminish when individuals are engaged in purposeful activities. The mind-body connection here is profound: By investing emotional energy in meaningful pursuits, we effectively shield our hearts from the detrimental impacts of chronic stress. Individuals who reported a high sense of purpose had significantly lower levels of C-reactive protein (CRP), a well-known marker of inflammation in the body.

Studies show that individuals with a strong sense of purpose have lower levels of pro-inflammatory cytokines and higher levels of oxytocin. This bonding hormone fosters resilience and social connection. This physiological shift explains why those who engage in purpose-driven activities, such as volunteering or mentoring, feel better emotionally and show measurable improvements in immune function and cardiovascular health.

Purpose is not just a nice idea, it is a physiological necessity. It sculpts our brain, optimizes our hormones, and extends our lifespan. It is the missing piece in modern health, the antidote to chronic stress, and the fuel for longevity. Whether through neuroscience, ancestral wisdom, or personal experience, one truth remains: A life driven by purpose is a life deeply lived.

Purpose: Betterment for Others.

Let us delve into a subtle yet significant distinction that can reshape our approach to personal growth: **getting better for others versus getting better than others.** In the whirlwind of modern society, it is easy to feel like we are competing in a relentless rat race, driven by the urge to outpace our peers, climb the social ladder, and bask in personal glory. But what if, instead of competing, we focused on harnessing our skills to serve those around us?

Drawing inspiration from the Hadzabe tribe and the Okinawan Japanese, each renowned for their interdependence, it is clear that true competence is not about standing out but about lifting everyone up. These groups prioritized their roles within their communities, striving to be the best versions of themselves, not for individual accolades but to contribute meaningfully to society.

For the Hadzabe, whether hunting big game or foraging for berries, developing skills maximizes benefits to the entire tribe, ensuring all share in the resources. Their pursuits are rooted in a shared purpose and a sense of belonging that fortifies the social fabric of their communities. This same spirit of cooperation in the Okinawans fosters "a reason for being." It emphasizes joy in what we do and honing talents that benefit others while enriching our lives.

Purpose: The Compass to Authentic Relationships

Connecting with our purpose charts a path for personal fulfillment and nurtures our relationships with others. In today's fast-paced world, where digital interactions often replace face-to-face connections, understanding and pursuing our inner purpose could be the key to bridging the gap between feeling isolated and genuinely connected. Discovering an inner purpose can be likened to finding a compass in the wilderness. This purpose provides direction, helping us make choices aligned with our core values and goals.

A clear purpose bolsters self-esteem and enhances self-image. We view ourselves more positively when we understand our place in the world and what drives us. Self-esteem is crucial for forming healthy relationships because it allows individuals to approach others with confidence and authenticity.

With a solid sense of purpose, individuals are less inclined to seek external gratification. This shift from outward validation to internal fulfillment transforms how we relate to people. Genuine connections are formed not from need but choice, fostering environments where relationships blossom authentically.

In America, loneliness is a growing concern. Although we can communicate with anyone, anywhere, we often fail to form deep, meaningful relationships. Studies show that the number of close confidants people have has declined, highlighting how digital tools might hamper us from developing genuine friendships.

The issue is a lack of social connections and a disconnect from ourselves. Forming genuine connections with others becomes challenging without clearly understanding who we are, our strengths, and our weaknesses. We align better with ourselves once we embrace our purpose, making us more relatable and open to others.

Self-discovery is crucial in cultivating purpose. Defining what truly matters to us and aligning our lives with these values creates a strong sense of self. This journey involves exploring personal strengths, passions, and the impact we wish to have. Clarity in purpose leads to genuine interactions. Studies indicated that those with a clear sense of purpose engage in more prosocial behaviors.

Once we connect with our purpose, we can extend this understanding to our interactions with others. Our personal growth allows us to form bridges with people sharing similar values or paths. This newfound connectedness is personally fulfilling and enriches community life by fostering mutual support and understanding.

Connecting with our inner purpose is pivotal in addressing the loneliness epidemic. It provides clarity and confidence, allowing us to form authentic connections with ourselves and others. Turning inward and understanding our life's compass enables us to navigate toward a future filled with meaningful relationships and community ties. It is time we move beyond digital ties and rekindle genuine connections, beginning with the one we have with ourselves.

The Ancestral Blueprint—Purpose Through Lineage and Craft

Somewhere deep in our bones, purpose is encoded. It is not a product of fleeting ambition or societal expectation, but a blueprint passed down through generations. In India, where my roots run deep, lineage is more than just genetics; it is a transmission of craft, knowledge, and dharma or life's purpose. Healers birth healers, artisans birth artisans, and storytellers pass on their words like heirlooms.

In my own family, this legacy was carved in wood. My ancestors were master woodworkers, sculpting not just furniture but art, their craft requiring equal parts vision, patience, and precision. If you have ever watched a true artisan at work, you know there is something almost meditative about it. Each stroke of the chisel, each careful cut, is not just mechanical labor but deep engagement, a merging of self and task. This is flow, the immersive state where skill and passion meet, and hours disappear in pursuing something greater than oneself.

Though I traded chisels for MRI scans, the essence of my lineage persists. Like woodworking, neuroradiology demands an ability to see beyond the surface, to recognize patterns where others see noise and patiently reconstruct what is hidden. I use the same focused attention my ancestors applied to carving a wooden masterpiece to read the human brain. Precision, patience, and the ability to reveal the unseen are not just skills, but an inheritance.

Purpose is not something we must manufacture from scratch, it is something waiting to be uncovered. What skills, passions, or impulses are encoded within you? What did your ancestors create, heal, build, or teach? Purpose is not about starting anew but remembering what was always there.

For those searching for purpose, the answer is often closer than they think. The clues are in childhood obsessions, family traditions, and moments when time ceases to exist.

The journey to purpose is not about seeking but *seeing* what has always been there. We are each born with an ancestral blueprint: a craft, a calling, a unique way of moving through the world. The challenge is not to find it but to *remember* it.

Primal Practices:

In our modern world, we often view purpose as an abstract concept, something to be found, like a hidden treasure. But purpose isn't discovered, it's cultivated. Just as a tree doesn't question whether it should grow, we are biologically wired for meaning. Neuroscience, evolutionary biology, and ancestral wisdom all point to purpose as an essential force for well-being. Below are seven primal, science-backed practices to develop purpose, enter flow, and awaken your ikigai.

1. Start Each Day with Intention
Before your feet hit the floor, take a moment to set your intentions. Ask yourself, "What do I want to accomplish today?" A clear purpose in the morning sets a positive tone for the day.

2. Practice Deep Work—Carve Out Focus Time
Multitasking is a myth. Neuroscientific studies confirm that deep work, that is, prolonged, uninterrupted focus—boosts myelin production and strengthens neural pathways. To cultivate purpose, set aside time for immersive work, whether writing, building, or creating.

3. Engage in a Craft—Use Your Hands
Whether it's woodworking, painting, or cooking, working with your hands taps into ancestral pathways of learning and mastery. MRI studies show that hands-on activities activate the sensorimotor cortex, engaging a deep neural feedback loop that

reinforces patience, attention, and problem-solving, all key purpose components.

4. Follow Curiosity—Trace the Origins of Your Fascination

Purpose is often hidden in what you lose track of time doing. What did you obsess over as a child? What makes hours feel like minutes? Identifying these clues can point you toward activities that naturally induce flow and meaning.

5. Engage in Flow Activities

Identify activities that make you lose track of time, those magical moments when you are completely absorbed. Whether painting, hiking, or problem-solving at work, regularly make time for these pursuits to enhance your sense of fulfillment.

6. Reflect on Your Skills

Each evening, jot down three things you did well that day. Recognizing your strengths nurtures self-esteem and reinforces your sense of purpose.

7. Tell Your Story—Make Sense of Your Journey

The human brain is wired for narrative. Studies on memory and cognition show that people who frame their life experiences within a coherent story experience less anxiety and greater clarity. Journaling, reflecting, and sharing your journey helps integrate past experiences into a purposeful trajectory.

Purpose isn't something we wait for; it's something we build through action, attention, and alignment. By engaging in these primal practices, you are not just living, you are thriving in sync with the very design of your biology. Find your flow, ignite your ikigai, and let your purpose evolve through the life you create every day.

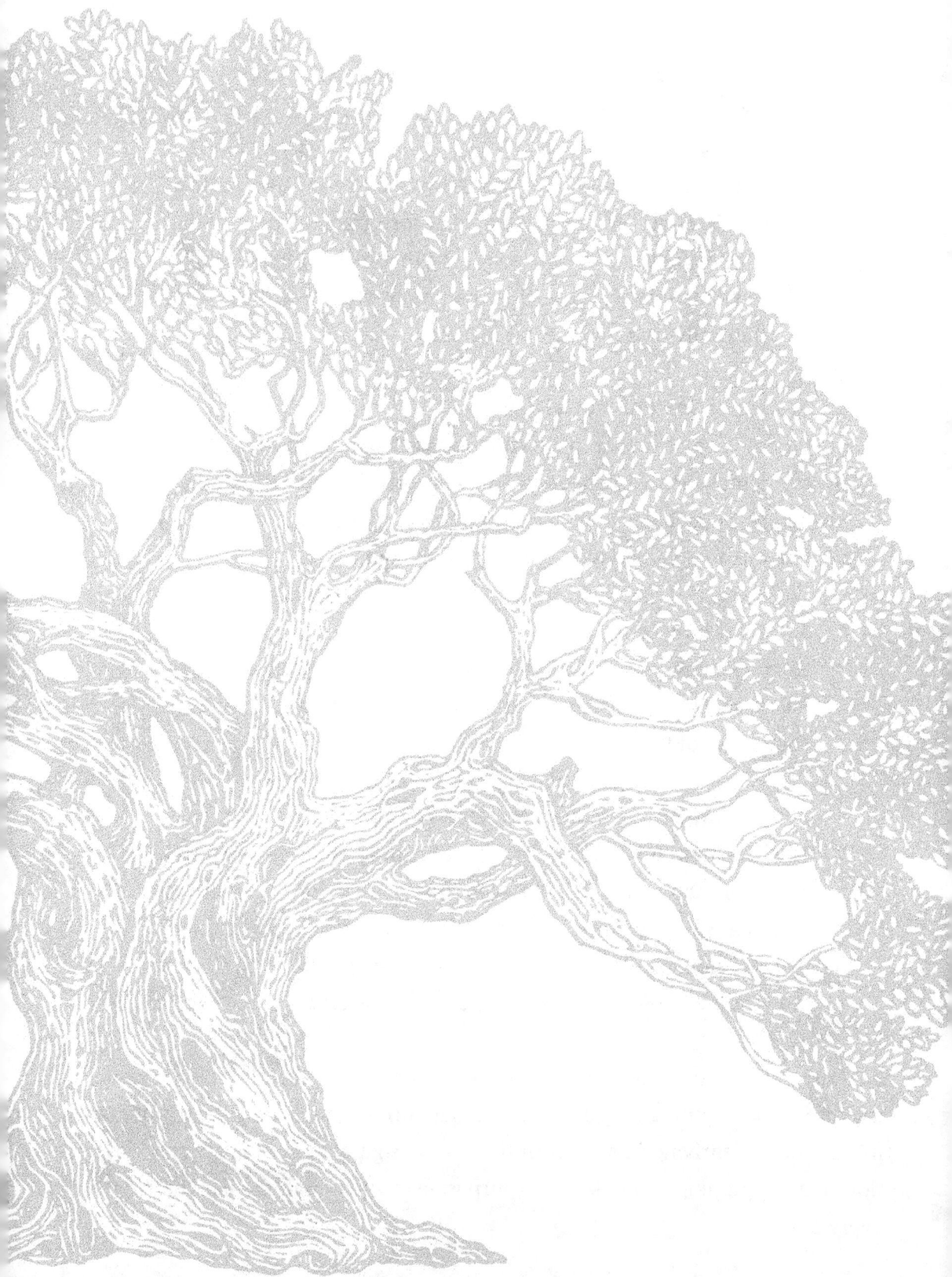

6

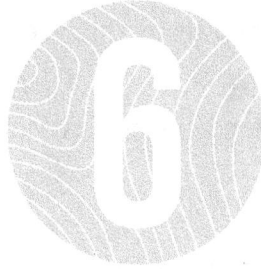

BEYOND SELF: BUILDING TRIBES AND PURPOSEFUL COMMUNITIES

"We are not meant to walk this path alone—our deepest purpose is woven into the lives we uplift, the tribes we build, and the legacy we leave behind."
— **Kavin Mistry, MD**

Ubuntu: The Power of We

The sun sank over the African savanna as the Hadza tribe gathered around a small fire. I watched as they passed around the evening's meal, not as a transaction, not keeping score, but as an unspoken contract of survival. No one hoarded. No one was left out. It wasn't about who had gathered the most tubers or who had landed the day's hunt. It was about something far more ancient: an unwritten code of life—Ubuntu. It's a concept as ancient as the land: **"Because we are, I am."**

Modern society worships self-sufficiency. We idolize the lone genius, the self-made billionaire, the rugged individualist. We post quotes about grinding on alone and cutting off people who "no longer serve us." But here, in the flickering glow of that fire, I saw the raw truth: Independence is an illusion.

Stephen Covey, in *The 7 Habits of Highly Effective People*, first introduced me to the concept of interdependence as he described the three stages of human development:

1. **Dependence** – The infant stage, where we rely on others for survival.

2. **Independence** – The adolescent illusion that we can do everything alone.

3. **Interdependence** – The mature realization that true success and fulfillment come from collaboration.

The modern world has glorified independence to the point of dysfunction. We celebrate the grind, the hustle, the lone wolf mentality. But the truth? The most successful people, the ones who *thrive*, aren't lone wolves. They're master collaborators. They know how to build, nurture, and sustain relationships. They don't just collect contacts, they cultivate *tribes*.

An African proverb sums it up best:

"If you want to go fast, go alone. If you want to go far, go together."

Life isn't a sprint; it's an endurance race. And if you want to finish strong, you need a pit crew. Your business partners. Your family. Your tribe.

In today's hyper-individualized world, learning to build an effective team is the real barometer of long-term success. Whether it's a mastermind group, a community, or a few trusted allies, your greatest assets aren't in your bank account or resume. They're sitting around your fire.

So, the real question is: Who's in your circle? And more importantly, who needs you in theirs?

Because at the end of the day, **I am because we are.**

Wired for Connection

"No man is an island." It's a cliché that's stood the test of time because it's profoundly true. We humans weren't designed to live in silos, scrolling endlessly through curated highlight reels on Instagram or chasing fleeting dopamine hits from likes and comments. Strip away the trappings of modern life, and what's left? The raw, primal truth: **We're wired for connection.** Our biology, our survival, and even our happiness depend on it.

But here's the kicker: Modern society has, in many ways, engineered connection out of our lives. We live in bigger houses but have smaller social circles. As discussed in the last chapter, we are digitally connected to more people, but we're lonelier than ever. The irony is hard to miss, and harder to live with.

Let's journey back to our community roots and examine why connection is not just a nice thing but a biological necessity.

Community and Longevity

One theme stands out in the grand story of human evolution: Our knack for working together. Tribal living was not just a choice but a survival advantage. By banding together, early humans created systems that ensured each member's well-being and success. This cooperative lifestyle wasn't just a way to survive; it was the formula for thriving.

Humans evolved to live in tribes, leveraging collective skills for mutual benefit. Everyone had a role in this context, whether you were a hunter scanning the horizon for game, a caregiver teaching the young, or a healer brewing tonics from nature's pharmacy. Each role was crucial for the tribe's endurance and triumph. This instinct for cooperation meant that no one was left behind. If a hunter failed one day, the group would still share resources to ensure everyone's survival. This collective resilience echoes through time, reminding us of the strength found in unity.

A fundamental yet often overlooked aspect of well-being is our profound need for community. This isn't just a touchy-feely concept; it's a vital component of our biology, deeply encoded in our DNA. Feeling part of a greater cause and connected to a community is essential for psychological health and physical well-being.

Through shared experiences and support networks, communities provide a social cushion and a boost to mental health by reducing feelings of isolation and despair. It's a buffer against life's storms, offering empathy, understanding, and companionship.

This concept is vividly illustrated in the study of Blue Zones, regions where people frequently live to be 100 years or older. Researchers found a common thread among these communities: robust social networks and daily social inter- actions. Whether it's sharing meals or participating in communal gatherings, sustained engagement with others plays a significant role in their extended lifespans. These connections provide emotional support and avenues for physi- cal activity and cognitive engagement, both vital for a thriving life.

Science underpins what many ancient cultures intuitively understand: **Social connections are a cornerstone of health and longevity.** This is why communal cultures, like the Hadzabe of Tanzania and the Okinawans of Japan, thrive. Their way of life isn't an accident, it's a masterclass in human biology.

The Hadzabe: A Case Study in Connection

The Hadzabe live in small, tightly knit groups, sharing food, responsibilities, and stories by the fire. Every individual plays a role in the community. Hunters bring back the game, and gatherers collect tubers and berries. Meals are shared equally. In this close-knit society, life isn't about individual gain but collective well-being. Daily interactions strengthen social bonds and foster mutual sup- port, vital threads in the tapestry of their existence. This daily interdependence fosters trust, reduces stress, and creates a sense of belonging.

For the Hadzabe, dancing and storytelling aren't extracurricular activities but fundamental aspects of life. They solidify bonds, ensure cultural transfer, and offer a shared sense of purpose. They remind us that designating time for community activities isn't a luxury but a necessity for emotional health.

The Hadzabe society operates on cooperative living, where leadership is rotational, and resources are shared. This system reflects deeply egalitarian values, fostering an environment where trust and communal effort supersede individual ambition.

The Hadzabe make decisions collectively, and everyone's input is valued. Resources from successful hunts are divided among tribe members, ensuring all benefit equally. This model highlights the benefits of living by the creed of communal cooperation instead of individual competition to create a harmony many of us crave in today's hyper-individualized world.

Anthropologists studying the Hadzabe have noted their remarkable health markers. They don't suffer from chronic stress or the loneliness epidemic plaguing modern society. Why? Because their lives are woven into the fabric of their community. They don't just survive together, they thrive.

Okinawan "Moai": Lifelong Support Systems

Thousands of miles away, on the Japanese island of Okinawa, lies another blueprint for community-driven health. Okinawans are among the world's longest-living people, with a disproportionately high number of centenarians.

What's their secret? A diet rich in vegetables and fish helps, but the real magic lies in their moai, close-knit social groups that provide lifelong emotional and financial support.

Okinawans don't just have friends; they have supportive networks. A moai is a group of five to ten people who commit to sticking together through thick and thin. They celebrate each other's joys, shoulder one another's burdens, and ensure no one ever feels alone. These lifelong groups create a fabric of security and friendship. Okinawans attribute much of their longevity to these social networks.

By integrating personal goals with communal objectives, Okinawans achieve what many struggle to experience: a deep sense of contentment and reduced stress. This shared purpose translates into the tangible health benefits of lowering cortisol levels (the notorious stress hormone) and reducing chronic inflammation, key players in numerous health conditions.

The Modern Loneliness Epidemic: What Went Wrong?

Now contrast these communal lifestyles with life in 2025. Many of us live in isolated bubbles, spending more time with screens than with people. We work long hours in individual cubicles or remote offices, grab dinner on the go, and scroll ourselves to sleep. The result? An epidemic of loneliness with devastating health consequences.

Today, our urban jungles and digital landscapes create "pseudo-communities." While we might be a click away from anyone globally, these digital connections often lack the depth and authenticity of true communal living. **We face an irony: We are infinitely "connected" yet deeply isolated.** Our digital lives, with notifications and tweets, skim the surface of what our ancestors experienced around campfires and shared meals.

The human brain is not designed for isolation. We are wired for connection, yet modern society has engineered a landscape of loneliness. Neuroscience has shown that chronic loneliness triggers the same brain regions as physical pain, a revelation that underscores our biological need for social bonds. Evolutionarily, being alone signified danger; separation from the tribe meant vulnerability to predators and scarce resources. Today, while saber-toothed threats no longer lurk in the shadows, social isolation has become the silent predator of modern life.

Loneliness is not just a feeling; it's a physiological stressor. Research indicates prolonged isolation elevates cortisol levels, increasing systemic inflammation and accelerating brain aging. Chronic loneliness is now recognized as a significant risk factor for cognitive decline and neurodegenerative diseases. Chronic social isolation is as lethal as smoking, yet society continues to treat it as an emotional inconvenience rather than a pressing health crisis.

If technology has allowed us to connect at the speed of light, why do so many people feel more disconnected than ever? The paradox of digital communication is that it offers the illusion of connection while starving us of its physiological benefits. Social media, messaging apps, and virtual interactions can never replace the biochemical magic of face-to-face engagement.

Dopamine, the neurotransmitter responsible for motivation and reward, fuels our addiction to social media. Every "like," comment, or notification provides a micro-hit of pleasure, reinforcing compulsive scrolling. But this dopamine-driven engagement is counterfeit currency; it lacks the oxytocin-rich bonding of real-world human interaction. True connection requires shared experiences, eye contact, laughter, and even synchronized heartbeats, none of which can be transmitted through a screen.

Furthermore, the digital world has hijacked our social instincts. Instead of fostering deep, meaningful relationships, we accept algorithmically curated feeds that reinforce superficial interactions. We scroll past human faces without registering them, replacing conversations with emojis and depth with brevity. This shift is not without consequences: **Studies show that increased screen time correlates with higher rates of depression, anxiety, and social withdrawal, particularly among younger generations.** In a world that glorifies hyper-independence, we must reframe interdependence not as a weakness but as an evolutionary superpower.

Research substantiates the benefits of fostering community ties. Studies on micro-communities have shown that small, intimate groups provide significant support against modern stressors, reducing feelings of isolation and increasing emotional resilience. These tight-knit circles can buffer against life's challenges, creating a safety net for mental and emotional well-being.

Conversely, excessive screen time and social media usage have been linked to negative health outcomes, including increased stress, anxiety, and feelings of loneliness. A meta-analysis found that individuals who spend more than two hours on social media each day report lower life satisfaction and higher levels of depression. While we may think we're connecting online, the quality of those interactions can often leave us feeling empty.

The Neuroscience of Community and Connection

Imagine sitting around a fire, sharing stories and laughter, or even enjoying a moment of shared silence. Biologically, it's more than the warmth you're feeling; this scene sparks the release of oxytocin, often called the "bonding hormone." When we share positive experiences with others, whether a deep conversation or a group effort toward a meaningful goal, oxytocin levels rise, reinforcing trust and social cohesion. This hormone doesn't just make us feel good; it actively reduces stress by counteracting cortisol, the body's primary stress hormone. In other words, strong relationships are not a luxury, they're a biological necessity.

Oxytocin works like social glue, reinforcing bonds, lowering stress levels, reducing inflammation, and even supporting your immune system. When you think of life-saving hormones, oxytocin probably doesn't make the list. But it should. It's the biochemical currency of connection. Want a longer, healthier life? Start with your relationships.

What does neuroscience have to say about our cooperative nature? Enter the world of mirror neurons, specialized brain cells that activate when we act and observe someone else doing the same thing we are doing. These neurons are the biological foundations of empathy and understanding, allowing us to learn through imitation and feel what others feel. When engaged in communal activities, these mirror neurons light up, signaling the brain to enjoy the shared experience. This physiological response underscores why group activities feel inherently rewarding; they're wired into our neurological framework.

Based on functional MRI studies, the human brain lights up in response to social interaction. The same neural networks activated when we experience personal joy also fire when we engage in acts of trust, belonging, and collective purpose. Our brains are not just built for connection, they *thrive* on it.

A key player in this social circuitry is the default mode network (DMN), a set of brain regions that govern introspection, empathy, and our sense of self in relation to others. When we interact with loved ones, collaborate with a team, or contribute to a greater cause, the DMN becomes more synchronized, strengthening neural pathways associated with emotional intelligence and long-term well-being.

Social engagement, especially warm, trusting relationships, also strengthens vagal tone (activity of the vagus nerve, key component of our parasympathetic system), enhancing our ability to regulate emotions and reducing systemic inflammation. People with higher vagal tone tend to be more resilient to stress, experience fewer chronic diseases, and even recover faster from illness. In contrast, isolation and chronic loneliness weaken vagal function, contributing to increased inflammation, higher cortisol levels, and a greater risk of anxiety and depression.

Put simply, meaningful connection is medicine.

Social bonds do more than shape our emotions; they physically rewire the brain. Thanks to neuroplasticity, the brain's ability to form and reorganize synaptic connections, strong relationships protect against cognitive decline and bolster mental resilience.

One of the most compelling pieces of evidence comes from Harvard's 75-year first-generation Study of Adult Development, which tracked participants' lives across decades. The conclusion? Wealth and success did not predict longevity. What did? The strength of their relationships. People with deep, fulfilling social ties not only lived longer but also maintained sharper cognitive function, lower rates of dementia, and greater overall life satisfaction.

From a neural perspective, we are designed to thrive in tribes. Our brains reward us for trust, collaboration, and shared purpose. The same systems that regulate stress, cognition, and even inflammation are wired to benefit from deep, meaningful social bonds.

In a world that often glorifies independence, our greatest strength lies in connection. Science affirms what we have intuitively known for millennia: Our health, happiness, and longevity are deeply intertwined with the relationships we nurture and the greater causes we serve.

Shared Purpose and Selfless Service

Something remarkable happens when people unite under a common cause such as restoring a local park, launching a green initiative, or organizing a neighborhood watch. Not only does the collective goal strengthen community bonds, but it also fuels personal fulfillment. It's that splendid paradox of giving; you receive so much more in return.

By stepping out of our individual bubbles and into a group's shared purpose, we tap into an infectious and invigorating energy. It's a feeling of being part of something greater than ourselves, which naturally builds resilience against life's challenges and boosts our mental health.

"Giving is receiving" isn't just poetic; it's backed by science. Engaging in altruistic activities such as volunteering can trigger a release of dopamine and serotonin, which keeps us happy and calm. This chemical cocktail translates into proactive behaviors, empowering individuals to lead healthier lives, and it's another line of defense against cognitive decline. Studies find that spending money on others lifts our spirits more than spending on ourselves. Talk about a win-win!

But the benefits don't stop there. **Regularly volunteering and partaking in altruistic activities have been linked to increased lifespan.** Researchers suggest that helping others activates reward-related brain regions and builds neural connections that can lead to a longer, healthier life.

Volunteering and participating in community-oriented efforts allow individuals to contribute their skills and knowledge while remaining socially connected. This social engagement is crucial. Research shows that individuals with strong social ties are better protected against cognitive decline. Frequent social interaction strengthens neural connections and enhances cognitive reserve, the brain's ability to compensate for damage.

The mechanics behind this connection are complex yet fascinating. Psychologists found that individuals with higher levels of purpose exhibited lower levels of neurodegenerative pathology in their brains. This suggests that a meaningful existence doesn't just improve life satisfaction but also fosters neurological health. By promoting a sense of purpose, we're not simply enriching our lives but actively fortifying our cognitive health against decline. Engaging in meaningful activities, whether through community service, honing a new skill, or advocating for a cause, is crucial for maintaining mental agility and a robust neurological health profile.

As we cultivate our purpose-driven lives, let's encourage those around us to seek their purpose. In a world that sometimes encourages looking out for oneself, remember that our purpose flourishes most brilliantly when shared. By uplifting one another, we create ripples of impact beyond ourselves, contributing to healthier, happier communities.

The Spirit of "Seva": Serving through Selflessness

Growing up in an Indian family, the concept of *samaj* (community) wasn't an abstract ideal but life itself. Every milestone, hardship, and celebration was a communal experience. You didn't just live for yourself; you lived for something greater. *Seva* (selfless service) was ingrained in the culture, not as an obligation but a source of fulfillment. Whether feeding stray animals before eating or donating time and resources to those in need, service was seen as a direct path to personal growth.

Seva translates to "selfless service," a practice that elevates personal growth through the art of giving without any expectation of reward. In our modern hustle and bustle, Seva serves as a timeless reminder of how intertwined our lives are and how profound the impact of service can be, both personally and communally.

When you think of Seva, imagine an act of kindness so pure that it transcends the giver-receiver dynamic. It's not counting favors or waiting for gratitude; it's about the simple joy of giving. Whether volunteering at a local charity, helping a neighbor with groceries, or spreading smiles at a community gathering, Seva is about heart-driven deeds with no strings attached.

In India, Seva is more than a term; it's a way of living interwoven into daily life. Temples often organize free meal services, providing food to needy people. These acts of giving nurture not just the physical body but also the spirit, reinforcing the belief that when we serve others, we enrich ourselves.

Engaging in Seva isn't just warm and fuzzy; it brings substantial psychological benefits. Acts of service activate a part of the brain associated with reward and pleasure, increasing dopamine levels, the "feel-good" neurotransmitter. Helping others helps you, too, by boosting your mood and fostering a sense of connectedness. Some call this the "helper's high." Whether checking on an elderly neighbor or assisting local organizations remotely, the essence remains the same: Contributing to the well-being of others enriches your own life.

By embedding selfless service into the core of community initiatives, we leverage its transformative power to address larger societal issues, whether tackling hunger, offering educational support, or creating safe spaces. After all, the heart of community isn't just where we live but how we live, together, in service, and harmony.

"In the joy of others lies our own." – **Pramukh Swami Maharaj**

Epigenetics of Bonding: Community as Medicine

Here's a fascinating nugget from the world of science: Positive social interactions may flip the genetic switches that help us cope with stress and bolster our immunity. In epigenetics, which studies how behaviors and environment can cause changes that affect how our genes work, interacting positively with others can upregulate genes associated with stress reduction and immune function. It's akin to having a natural pharmacist at your beck and call, dispensing wellness instead of pills.

This phenomenon highlights the power of community. Each warm smile or comforting hug isn't just a fleeting moment; it's a mini-therapy session for your genes, encouraging them to express themselves in ways that enhance resilience and health.

For the Hadzabe, living outdoors in constant communion with their environment and each other is not merely a lifestyle choice; it's a health necessity.

The tranquil atmosphere and consistent social interaction lower stress markers in these natural settings. This reminds us how far we've drifted from our roots and how reconnecting with nature and each other could be the key to reducing stress and enhancing our well-being.

Over in Okinawa, the famed centenarians live out another testament to the power of connection—communal meals that nourish both body and soul. Sharing food isn't just about sustenance; it's also about reinforcing relationships and fostering a sense of belonging. Studies, like those supporting the Blue Zone findings, show that these shared experiences lead to better nutrient absorption and a lower incidence of overeating. When chatter is a side dish to your meal, you may eat less and enjoy more!

The benefits of collective healing aren't new to therapists who see the transformative power of group therapy. Research shows that individuals in group settings often experience heightened healing from trauma and improved mental health compared to one-on-one therapeutic endeavors. Shared stories and support instill a sense of understanding and belonging that accelerates recovery.

The verdict is clear: Human connection is much more than a social nicety. It's a healing balm with profound mental, emotional, and physical health implications. Whether we are looking at epigenetics, the healing power of nature, or Okinawan shared meals, the message is resoundingly hopeful: **We heal best when we heal together.** Let's cultivate spaces where our collective stories and shared laughter become powerful medicine.

Limbic Resonance: The Wi-Fi of Human Connection

Imagine stepping into a room and feeling an immediate sense of upliftment; the chatter is animated, the laughter infectious, and the atmosphere electric with energy. Or perhaps it's a serene meditation circle where tranquility seems to fill every corner. These experiences transcend mere subjective responses; they're vivid manifestations of a captivating biological phenomenon known as limbic resonance. This concept highlights the remarkable interplay between our emotions and those of the company we keep.

So, what's at play here? Enter the domain of limbic resonance, a term that describes the remarkable ability of our limbic system, our brain's emotional epicenter, to sync with others'. It is the process of emotional contagion where our moods are both influential and influenced. Within these interactions, our nervous systems effectively exchange signals, setting off an emotional frequency that others intuitively tune into.

Picture the limbic system as an invisible emotional Wi-Fi, connecting everyone within its range. We're wired for social connection, so we're inherently equipped to resonate harmoniously with the emotions of friends, family, and even strangers. This resonance is the glue that fosters empathy, rapport, and social cohesion.

Why is this important? Thanks to the miraculous feature of limbic resonance, our communities profoundly impact our neurobiology.

Shared Moods and Health

Just as smiling can spread like wildfire through a room, so can emotions like anxiety or joy. This interconnectedness means that our collective emotional states are more than just mood enhancers; they are architects of our mental and physical well-being. Positive group interactions can lower stress hormones like cortisol and boost feel-good chemicals such as serotonin and dopamine.

Feeling Calmer Together

Have you ever noticed how stepping into a yoga class or attending a harmonious family dinner can immediately instill calmness? That's no fluke. Our brains naturally mirror the emotional tenor of the group, guiding us into a calmer state when surrounded by joyful and relaxed people.

Enhanced Learning and Inspiration

Limbic resonance can supercharge our learning and creativity when we're part of an engaged, dynamic group. It's the secret explaining why brainstorming sessions ignite novel ideas or motivational seminars rekindle passion. In these settings, the collective energy acts as a catalyst for cognitive breakthroughs.

The ripple effects of limbic resonance extend far and wide, subtly shaping everything from personal well-being to professional productivity. Consider workplace morale: An enthusiastic leader can elevate the team by radiating positivity, while his perpetually stressed counterpart risks inadvertently spreading stress by contagion.

Understanding limbic resonance offers profound insights. It tells us that our choices about whom we engage with are significant, both philosophically and biologically. As community architects, we possess the power to construct environments suffused with positive emotion, yielding tangible benefits for everyone involved.

We foster more resilient and connected communities by mindfully cultivating spaces encouraging healthy emotional contagion. Elevating our shared emotional state enhances individual happiness and reinforces the social fabric binding us together. Through intentional choices of positivity, connection, and community, we become the architects of our emotional ecosystems, orchestrating symphonies of shared joy and collective well-being.

The Road Ahead: Rekindling Our Tribal Roots

The sun sets differently when you're not watching it alone. There's something about sharing a moment, be it a meal, a laugh, or even a struggle, that amplifies its meaning. We were never meant to go through life in isolation. And yet, modern society has subtly convinced us that self-sufficiency is the pinnacle of success. We've traded village fires for screen glow, elders' wisdom for algorithmic YouTube feeds, and communal survival for individual hustle.

But **longevity isn't just about eating well, exercising, or optimizing biomarkers. It's about connection. Social isolation is the modern-day equivalent of malnutrition.**

The science of connection runs deep. Ever notice how stress feels lighter when shared or how joy expands in the presence of others? That's biology at work. Our ancestors didn't just tolerate community; they relied on it for survival. Today, we need it just as much, even if our saber-toothed threats have been replaced by chronic stress and existential angst.

Every interaction, every hug, every moment of shared purpose leaves molecular signatures on our genes. The Hadzabe and Okinawans, these long-lived communities, don't just eat better or move more. They belong. When you are embedded in a network of mutual support, your body knows it. It shifts from a survival state to a thriving state. This is why elders in Okinawa don't retire to solitude, they become mentors.

Community isn't just a feel-good idea. It's a biological imperative. When we connect, we thrive. When we isolate, we wither. The Hadzabe and Okinawans aren't relics of the past; they're reminders of what we've lost and what we can reclaim.

The Real Measure of a Life Well-Lived

While urbanization and digital networks might reshape how we interact, the core principles of tribal living, such as empathy, cooperation, and collective endurance, remain unchanged. It's time to reawaken that tribal spirit and infuse our pseudo-communities with authentic depth and connectivity. These insights compel us to reflect on our connections and encourage us to foster genuine, fulfilling relationships because a vibrant life hinges on the company we share.

Ultimately, the question isn't how long we live but how connected we live. The key to longevity isn't found in a lab; it's found around the fire, at the dinner table, in the simple act of showing up for each other. Because at the deepest level of our biology, community isn't optional. It's survival. It's healing. It's home.

The path forward is clear. To design a truly primal life, we must reweave ourselves into the tapestry of community. In the end, the greatest purpose we can serve is each other.

Primal Practices:

1. Find Your People, and Invest in Them

Humans aren't meant to be lone wolves. Whether it's a mastermind group, a fitness crew, a book club, or your extended family, cultivate relationships that fuel you. Friendships aren't just for fun; they're a biological necessity. Strong social bonds reduce stress hormones, increase longevity, and make life much more enjoyable.

2. Prioritize Face Time (No, Not the App)

Texting is not talking. Zoom calls are not hugs. Your biology knows the difference. Real human connection—eye contact, touch, laughter—triggers oxytocin, the ultimate feel-good, stress-busting hormone. Meet for coffee, take a walk with a friend, or throw a dinner party. Your nervous system will thank you.

3. Break Bread Together, Often

Every culture has food at the center of gatherings. Shared meals strengthen bonds, build trust, and create lasting memories. Plan weekly dinners, host potlucks, or just eat with others instead of solo-scrolling through your phone. Longevity studies show that communal eating leads to healthier, happier lives.

4. Build Your Moai—Your Tribe for Life

Okinawans have a concept called Moai, a close-knit group that supports each other through life's ups and downs. Who's in your Moai? Cultivate deep friendships, commit to showing up for each other, and foster a support network that strengthens over time. Health isn't just about diet and exercise, it's about who has your back.

5. Align With a Cause Bigger Than Yourself

Volunteering, mentoring, and contributing to something greater than yourself isn't just good for the world, it's essential for you. Studies show that having a sense of purpose extends lifespan and increases happiness. Get involved in community service, environmental activism, or supporting a local initiative. Purpose is a primal fuel.

6. Create Rituals That Anchor Connection

Modern life is chaotic. Rituals create structure and deepen bonds. Weekly game nights, morning workouts with a friend, group meditation, or even a Friday night phone call with your best friend are little traditions that keep relationships strong and your primal circuitry firing.

7. Choose Interdependence Over Isolation

Modern culture glorifies independence, but real resilience comes from interdependence. The Hadzabe, the Amish, and the longest-living communities in the world all thrive on strong communal ties. The Indian concept of samaj (community) reminds us that life isn't about isolated achievement but about shared purpose. Prioritize relationships over transactions. Engage in service without expecting returns. Find meaning in contributing to something beyond yourself.

The Bottom Line: We don't need to abandon modern life and retreat to the wilderness to reclaim our tribal instincts. We just need to be intentional about connection. Share meals, hug often, laugh together, serve a cause, and build your tribe. **The quality of your life is, and always has been, measured by the strength of your connections.**

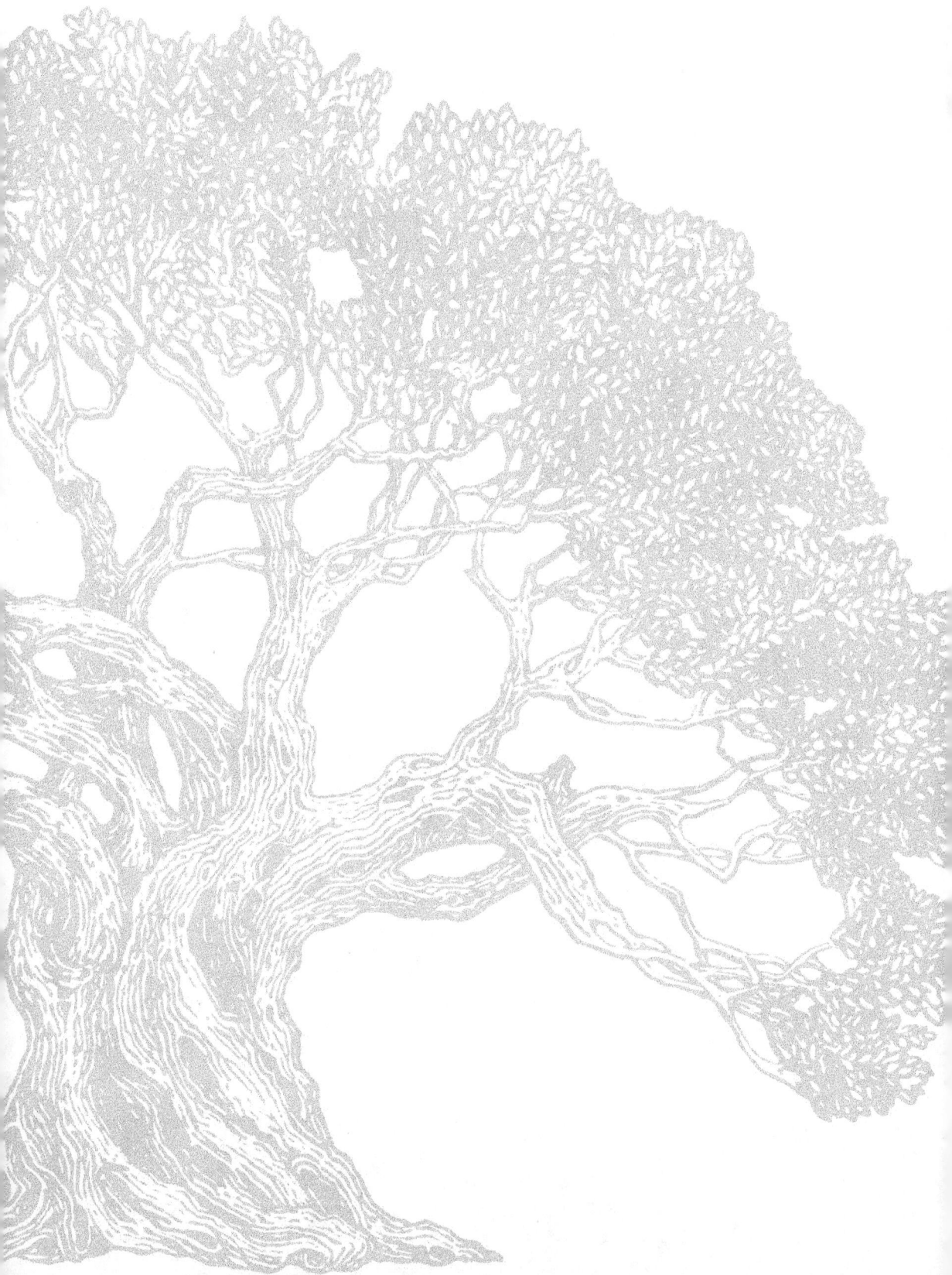

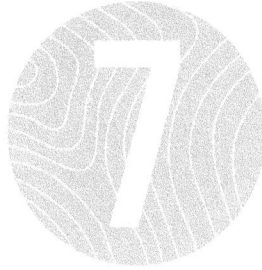

COSMIC CONNECTION: EMBRACING THE FINITE WITHIN THE INFINITE

"We are perishable, yet we live among the stars. We are finite, yet we touch the infinite."
– Carl Sagan.

As the sun dipped low over the horizon, casting a golden hue across the sprawling savanna, a young Hadzabe hunter stood poised, every muscle taut with intention. His eyes methodically surveyed a herd of wildebeest grazing peacefully nearby, oblivious to the ritual significance of their existence that day. This wasn't just another hunt but a sacred moment leading him toward adulthood, the Epeme ceremony.

In Hadzabe culture, the term "Epeme men" is reserved for those who have slain large game, typically in their early twenties. It's a rite of passage that carves the first real milestones of manhood, bestowing honor and privilege. Only these men are allowed to consume specific parts of prized game: warthogs, giraffes, buffalo, wildebeest, and even lions. Each kill signifies personal achievement and maintains a delicate balance within the tribe, showcasing the intrinsic connection between life and death.

As the hunter observed the herd, his skills honed by generations of tradition came alive. He identified the older wildebeests, understanding their vulnerabilities; they would provide the easiest target. Yet, this wasn't just about the physical act of hunting. He perhaps grasped the deeper essence of the cycle of life, how his successful hunt would forge his passage into manhood, a process that required the sacrifice of an aged beast.

This awareness mirrored the profound philosophy that underpins the Hadzabe way of life. **Death, in its raw truth, gives birth to life anew.** The hunter felt a calmness wash over him as he contemplated his role in this cosmic circle, a recognition that one day, just like the animals he hunted, he, too, would serve as a vessel for new experiences to flourish. There was no unrealistic illusion of immortality here; instead, a profound understanding of the finite nature of existence shaped his worldview.

This reverence for mortality invokes peace rather than fear, crafting a mental framework that amplifies appreciation for every moment. He understood that, in the face of death, true vitality emerges. Life's beauty lies in its brevity, compelling us to cherish each breath and relationship.

Reflecting on these themes brings to mind one of my all-time favorite films: *Bicentennial Man (Columbus, 1999)*, starring Robin Williams. The story encapsulates the touching narrative of a robot who outlives everyone he loves. As time drags on, he yearns to experience mortality, craving the entirety of the human experience, including death itself. When he is finally granted his wish, he passes away with a smile, fully embracing his life and the connections he formed.

In seeking longevity, we often overlook its more significant purpose: to live not just long but richly, intertwined with family and community. No one truly seeks to outlive their loved ones, including children. Instead, **we must reframe our approach to mortality into a space that offers us strength, a foundation from which we can live profoundly and purposefully.**

As we delve into the concept of existential health, this chapter will unfold the wisdom embedded in these cycles of life, the lessons derived from embracing mortality, and how they can guide us toward a balanced and fulfilling existence.

Together, let's explore the intricate dance between life and death and the profound beauty that emerges from understanding and accepting our finite nature.

The Paradox of Mortality and Longevity

"The greatest tragedy is getting to the end of your life and realizing you never truly lived." – **Sadhguru**

In our hustle and bustle, we operate under the illusion of endless tomorrows, convincing ourselves with "perhaps next time" or "one of these days." Mortality rarely crosses our minds as we squirrel away promotions, possessions, and victories for some future that never seems to arrive.

The ultimate paradox is that we operate with a finite mindset when we think we have an infinite life. We get caught in the web of a win-lose game, and life winds up being purely transactional. When you finally see life's finite nature, transformation occurs. You transition to playing an infinite game, where meaning eclipses ambition and experiences dwarf trophies. Everything changes once you understand that we all come into this world with nothing and leave with nothing.

Envision operating with an infinite mindset, recognizing that we all cross the same finish line. There is no winner in the longevity race. Simon Sinek explores this beautifully in *The Infinite Game*. It's not about winning an argument with your partner but deepening your relationship gracefully as you age. It's not about your children reaching Ivy League milestones but nurturing them to become compassionate individuals who contribute to society. For me, as an academic physician, it's not about clocking in for a paycheck but raising the next generation of doctors who embody both skill and empathy. True fulfillment comes when you go beyond making more of yourself every day and work on the legacy you will leave behind.

In our pursuit of extending lifespan, we sometimes forget the essence of truly living. When the finiteness of life is truly comprehended, you selectively invest your time and energy into things that bear significance. **Health transforms from something you pursue for yourself to something you ensure for the shared joy of experiences with loved ones.** No one needs to twist your arm to hit the gym when staying healthy for your spouse is at stake.

Otherwise, you risk being fit but not fulfilled, financially free but not content, famous yet hollow. We all know of celebrities trapped in this paradox; their stories echo tragic headlines. Social media perpetuates this quest for external significance yet rarely addresses our inherent desire for internal fulfillment.

Paradoxically, it's death that gives life its meaning. If we lived forever, moments would lose their magic, urgency, and beauty. When immortality feels certain, life turns transactional. However, if you knew you only had 24 hours, every interaction would change. You would savor each moment.

As we age, we tend to fear death so intensely that we become paralyzed, never truly living. Yet, embracing the finite within the infinite allows us to transcend fear. **Death doesn't diminish life; it defines it, shades it, gives it weight and texture.** Amid the uncertainty, we're invited to view our lives with the gentle knowledge that our limited time makes time precious. As we engage with this profound truth, we unlock a profound appreciation for life's fleeting, ever-beautiful moments.

Embracing Finiteness to Live Fully

As we ponder the dance of life and death, we learn that mortality isn't just an endpoint, it's a profound teacher guiding us toward enriched living. Understanding our finite nature is not a morbid exercise but a powerful catalyst for making choices that enhance our longevity and quality of life. **Oddly enough, mortality can serve as a wellspring for wellness.**

Existential psychology illuminates the surprising benefits of confronting our own mortality. Individuals who accept and embrace their finite nature often report making healthier life decisions. For instance, they smoke less, exercise more, and maintain improved diets. It seems that experiencing the reality of a finite existence encourages choices that add flavor and health to one's days.

The implications extend further. Acknowledging mortality has been linked to reduced stress levels, which, in turn, lower inflammation and boost longevity markers. Gazing into the transient nature of life removes the veil of stress, allowing us to focus on what truly matters and enhancing our well-being on a cellular level.

Sacred Ash: Lessons from India

This transformative perspective resonates with ancient wisdom, as seen in various cultures. Take, for example, the saints in India who cover themselves in ash, symbolizing their embrace of mortality and life's fleeting nature. Ash, a stark reminder that we begin and end as dust, is worn with pride, encouraging a vigorous, passionate approach to life.

This symbolic act instills a deep respect for the impermanence of existence, urging individuals to live with energetic intention. For these saints, and perhaps for all of us, it's not about living forever but living fully, acknowledging life's inherent brevity, and savoring each moment.

This practice is not isolated to spiritual realms; it offers a metaphor applicable to us. Embracing our finite nature encourages a life marked by deliberate choices and mindful presence, fostering a fulfilling journey no matter the length.

Cosmic Connection: From Neurons to Galaxies

As a neuroradiologist, I often find myself enmeshed in the intricate workings of the human brain, the labyrinthine structures and vibrant pathways that reveal the stories of our thoughts, emotions, and experiences. The brain's natural inclination to seek patterns, meaning, and connection never ceases to amaze me. It's as if our minds are wired to search through the chaos for coherence, desperately trying to string together the fragmented pieces of existence into a comprehensible narrative.

The Power of Cosmic Awe

There's something deeply moving about gazing up at a starlit sky, the vast expanse that suggests the enormity of the universe and our humble place within it. This phenomenon, often referred to as cosmic awe, has garnered scientific interest. Studies indicate that experiencing awe can lower inflammation, improve mental well-being, and even enhance feelings of connectedness.

The beauty of this experience lies in how it diminishes the ego, coaxing us to confront the colossal reality beyond our everyday lives. In this state, we realize how our trifles pale in comparison to the grandeur of the universe. This perspective enhances our resilience against life's challenges as we understand that our struggles become mere ripples in the grand ocean of existence.

On a deeper level, the yearning for connection to this cosmic arena resonates with a universal truth: Beneath the layers of individuality, we seek to reconnect with the singular energy that binds us all. Throughout life, we often chase after distinctions, endeavors that carve out our specialness in the world, but that journey can cloak us in isolation. **Within each of us lies a core desire for unity with the cosmos, a piece of our being that seeks to understand where our finite lives fit within this vast and infinite universe.**

In his seminal work, *Man's Search for Meaning*, Viktor Frankl described the "existential vacuum," the feeling of emptiness and meaninglessness that arises when we lose sight of our purpose. This vacuum often arises when we obsessively focus on our distinctions, accolades, or compulsions, forgetting that life's richness is deeply connected with ourselves and the universe.

As we stand on the threshold of our existence, grappling with questions of meaning within an infinite cosmos, let's remember to seek individuality and embrace the beauty of unity. Our mind craves to weave patterns, our spirit yearns for connection, and we free ourselves from the shackles of isolation by recognizing our oneness with this vast universe.

The Health Benefits of a Cosmic Perspective

When we contemplate the vastness of the universe, we feel a sense of humility, but also wonder, about our place within it. Approximately 13.8 billion years old, the universe has witnessed countless stars' birth and death, galaxies' formation, and unimaginable cosmic events. In stark contrast, the average human lifespan hovers around 80 years, a mere blink in the cosmic timeline.

If the average human lives around 80 years in a 13.8-billion-year-old universe, our existence occupies approximately 0.00000058% of that timeline. In relatable terms, **if the universe's entire history were compressed into a single calendar year, human life would amount to only a few seconds before midnight on December 31st.**

This perspective can be humbling. While our lives may feel important and urgent, cosmic reality prompts us to ask fundamental questions about meaning and legacy. Are we spending our short burst of time collecting treasures or nurturing relationships? Are we chasing accolades in the fleeting race of life or embracing the simple connection that binds us to the universe?

Engaging with this perspective invites us to elevate our focus beyond individual accomplishments toward something more significant: Our shared humanity and the impact we can have in the brief moments we are given. It compels us to cherish life and foster connections, not only with each other but with the essence of existence echoed throughout the cosmos.

Embracing a cosmic perspective can enhance our physical and mental well-being. When we quiet the noise of daily stresses and invest our energy in meaningful connections and activities, we promote better mental health and reduce the risks of chronic illnesses. Moreover, by adopting an expansive view of life, we cultivate a mindset that embraces change and uncertainty, a particularly beneficial quality as we age. Engaging in reflective practices, like stargazing or pondering our place in the universe, can stimulate introspection and gratitude, further magnifying our psychological resilience.

Embracing Oneness: The Eastern Philosophy of Unity

In the ancient tales of the Buddha, a powerful story has reverberated through the centuries, retaining its wisdom and relevance even today. Upon welcoming new monks into the fold of monkhood, the Buddha would often send them to the cremation grounds, a striking initiation ritual designed not to shock or disgust but to remind them of life's impermanence. There, amidst the crackling flames and wafting smoke of burnt offerings, the monks would witness the bodies of their fellow beings being released back to the universe. It was a sobering experience, yet one steeped in profound purpose.

The intent behind this practice was simple yet impactful: to instill a sense of urgency and perspective in the hearts of the initiates. By closely observing the inevitable journey of life's physical form back to the elements, monks learned the essential truth of detachment, not just from the body itself, but from the fleeting thoughts and emotions that can entrap us. This initiation was the first step in their spiritual journey, encouraging them to seek a grander connection with existence, transcending the ephemeral and embracing the eternal.

The Concept of Oneness

This philosophy of oneness, deeply rooted in Eastern thought, teaches us that all life is interconnected and a manifestation of the same universal energy. Separation, often perceived as reality, is merely an illusion. **Understanding this interconnectedness fosters compassion and empathy, qualities that allow us to recognize ourselves in others and appreciate the collective experience of living.**

Indian philosophies in particular embody this concept. The ancient texts encourage us to view ourselves not as isolated beings but as integral threads woven into the vast fabric of existence. Through practices we have covered that cultivate mindfulness, such as yoga, pranayama (breath control), and compassion meditations, we can realign ourselves with this profound truth, inhibiting the sense of separation that modern life often imposes.

Compassion meditation, which focuses on cultivating feelings of love and kindness toward ourselves and others, fosters emotional healing and creates a biological shift. Practicing compassion has been linked to improved immune response and lower cortisol levels, another reflection of how inner transformations lead to outer well-being.

Similarly, the emerging field of epigenetics highlights how our lifestyle choices, such as practicing mindfulness, can influence gene expression, turning on or off the switches that determine health outcomes. This correspondence between Eastern traditions and Western scientific discoveries validates the age-old belief that wellness extends beyond the physical, intricately weaving together mind, body, and spirit.

The story of the Buddha sending monks to the cremation grounds poignantly reminds us of life's impermanence and urges us toward a deeper connection with our existence. By recognizing our oneness with others and the universe, we can transcend the boundaries of separation imposed by our busy lives. Embracing practices grounded in compassion, mindfulness, and unity enriches our lives and significantly impacts our health.

The Interconnectedness of All Things

One truth emerges across ancient traditions and modern science: Everything is connected. This isn't just a feel-good philosophy; it's a fundamental reality woven into the very fabric of existence. Life moves from the vast cosmos to the tiniest subatomic particles in a dynamic, interwoven dance.

Eastern philosophies (Hinduism, Buddhism, Taoism) have long taught that we're not isolated beings floating through an indifferent universe. Instead, we're threads in an intricate tapestry, each of us bound to one another and to nature itself. Modern science, particularly quantum physics and ecology, echoes this wisdom in striking ways.

Think about it. The air you breathe was once exhaled by ancient forests. The iron in your blood was forged in the heart of distant stars. Life isn't just connected, it's a seamless flow of energy and matter, continuously recycled through time and space.

Even at the tiniest levels, science reveals a deep interconnectedness. Take quantum entanglement, one of the strangest phenomena in physics. Imagine you have two tiny particles that become "entangled." No matter how far apart they move, even if one is on Earth and the other is light-years away, when you change one, the other responds instantly. It's as if they're invisibly linked, communicating across space with no apparent delay. Einstein called this "spooky action at a distance." Scientists don't fully understand how it works, but it suggests a hidden unity underlying all things.

This isn't just happening at the quantum level. It's everywhere in nature. The mycelium network beneath a forest floor allows trees to "talk" to each other, sharing nutrients and warnings about environmental threats. Bees and flowers co-evolved in a perfect exchange of sustenance. The human microbiome, trillions of bacteria living inside us, is essential to our health and well-being. Life thrives on cooperation, not isolation.

The message?

Nothing exists in a vacuum. Everything—from the atoms in our cells to the ecosystems that sustain us—is part of an intricate, self-sustaining web.

When we embrace this oneness, something shifts. Studies show that people who feel connected to a community, nature, or a sense of purpose experience less anxiety and depression. Practices like meditation and mindfulness help us tune into this connection. When you meditate, you're not just calming your mind, you're tapping into something larger. You begin to sense the pulse of life within and around you, dissolving the illusion of separateness.

Living with Oneness

So, how do we bring this awareness into everyday life? Simple:

- **Practice presence.** Slow down. Feel the ground beneath your feet, the rhythm of your breath, the sun on your skin.

- **Act with kindness.** Every interaction sends ripples through the web of life. Choose to send waves of compassion.

- **Stay curious.** The more we learn about the natural world, the more we see how deeply intertwined we are with it.

We are not isolated dots in the universe; we are brushstrokes in a master-piece, chords in a grand symphony, and notes in an endless melody. The more we recognize this, the richer and more meaningful life becomes.

Because in the end, oneness isn't something to seek; it's something we already are.

The Legacy of Creation

In the bustling workshop of my family's history, every groove and grain of wood tells the story of a lineage of artisans who sculpted more than just furniture; they sculpted meaning. The Mistry family name carries the weight of creation, each piece a lasting testament to craftsmanship, patience, and the pursuit of excellence.

In an era obsessed with speed and instant gratification, the slow, deliberate act of making something tangible is a form of quiet rebellion. This isn't just nostalgia talking. Science confirms that working with our hands, whether through woodworking, painting, sculpting, or even gardening, does more than produce art. It regenerates the mind, rewires the brain, and fosters resilience.

The Neuroscience of Craftsmanship

Picture the rhythmic motion of a chisel carving into wood, the fluid dance of a brush across the canvas, or the firm yet delicate shaping of clay. These acts of creation aren't merely aesthetic pursuits; they are workouts for the brain. Neuroscience tells us that hands-on activities stimulate neuroplasticity (the brain's ability to form new neural connections) enhancing cognitive flexibility, memory, and emotional regulation.

The brain fires synchronously across multiple regions whenever we take on a creative challenge. Woodworking, for example, isn't just about carving; it requires spatial reasoning, fine motor coordination, and problem-solving, each engaging different neural networks. This dynamic activation strengthens cognitive pathways, making the mind more adaptable and resilient.

Studies show that engaging in creative work reduces cortisol levels by alleviating stress and lowering the risk of neurodegenerative diseases. The process also triggers the release of dopamine, our brain's natural reward chemical, reinforcing motivation and emotional well-being. The more we create, the more we cultivate a cognitive reserve as a buffer against aging and mental decline.

Perhaps the most fascinating aspect of creativity is the flow state, a deeply immersive experience where time seems to vanish. When fully absorbed in a creative task, the brain enters a state of heightened focus, synchronizing thought and action with an almost meditative result. This state has been linked to increased productivity, greater life satisfaction, and even enhanced problem-solving abilities.

Building a Mental and Emotional Legacy

Engaging in craftsmanship is more than just a means of self-expression. It's also an existential anchor. It fosters presence, intention, and connection to something larger than ourselves. When we create, we aren't just shaping objects; we are shaping the mental landscapes of future generations.

I still run my hands over furniture crafted by my ancestors more than a century ago. These pieces have weathered time, bearing witness to historical transitions, family milestones, and personal narratives etched in their grain. They remind me that creation isn't just about the present, it's about contributing to a lineage of meaning.

Leaving a legacy isn't about grand gestures or monumental achievements. It's about embedding purpose into our daily work through supporting causes, designing, or investing in people. It's about resisting distraction in favor of deep, meaningful engagement. In doing so, we construct something lasting in the physical world and fortify our minds, leaving behind a blueprint for future generations to follow.

The Call to Create

I urge you to embrace creative outlets as a way of connecting with your mortality while leaving a tangible legacy. For it is in crafting something enduring that we find personal fulfillment and contribute to something greater than ourselves.

Pick up a chisel, a pen, a microphone, anything that allows you to create with intention. Not just for productivity but for the sake of your brain, your well-being, and your place in the unfolding narrative of human creativity. This book is my pursuit to that end.

We witness the magic of leaving a lasting imprint when we create with intention, whether by crafting a physical object, raising a child, or supporting a cause from the ground up. It's not just about the finished product but the stories, connections, and memories forged along the way.

Legacy is not an endpoint; it is a continuum, a ripple effect of creation that stretches far beyond our lifetime. In crafting something enduring, we affirm the richness of our existence, forging connections between past, present, and future. Let's honor this tradition, one mindful creation at a time.

Grace vs. Gravity: The Dance of Vitality

Imagine life as a grand ballet, where two opposing forces choreograph our existence: grace and gravity. From a scientific perspective, these forces aren't just metaphors. They're grounded in principles that govern health, vitality, and longevity. In *Primal Health Design*, understanding and harnessing these forces is key to optimizing our well-being.

Gravity: The Force of Decay and Aging

Let's start with gravity, the ever-constant pull towards entropy, that inevitable tendency of systems to fall into disorder over time. In the realm of biology, gravity manifests as aging, degeneration, and cellular breakdown, a relentless dance partner determined to slow our strides.

1. **Aging and Cellular Decline:** As we age, our cells experience senescence, losing their youthful ability to divide and regenerate.

2. **Oxidative Stress:** Think of free radicals as rogue dancers

causing oxidative damage to cells, proteins, and DNA, accelerating the aging process.

3. **Muscle Atrophy and Posture:** Quite literally, gravity pulls us downward, leading to muscle weakening and bone loss, especially if we remain inactive.

4. **Metabolic Slowdown:** A sedentary lifestyle is like sitting out the dance entirely, amplifying gravity's effect and dragging us into decline.

Unaddressed, gravity is like a rock rolling downhill, determined to erode our vibrance.

Grace: The Force of Renewal and Vitality

Enter grace, the creative counterforce that draws its strength from renewal and vitality, urging us to rise above gravity's pull. Grace promotes adaptability and homeostasis, showcasing the body's incredible capacity for self-rejuvenation:

1. **Neuroplasticity:** With each new step and twist, the brain forms new connections, counteracting decline by nurturing learning and resilience.

2. **Autophagy:** Grace fuels the body's spring cleaning (autophagy) where fasting, exercise, and sleep encourage the removal of cellular debris and promote renewal.

3. **Resistance Training and Hormesis:** Exercises like weightlifting and hill climbing are metaphors for dancing against gravity, building strength, resilience, and hormonal balance.

4. **Mind-Body Practices:** Meditation and mindfulness act like a

gentle hand on our back, reducing stress and activating parasympathetic activity, thereby promoting balance.

5. **Telomere Preservation:** Menus that feature nourishing
nutrition, regular exercise, and restful sleep help maintain
telomere length, a key to cellular vitality.

Grace is akin to soaring on an updraft: an intentional force that lifts us
upward through deliberate alignment with the natural laws of health.

Integrating the Two Forces

At the center of *Primal Health Design,* vitality emerges from cultivating practices
that harness grace to counteract gravity. When we flow with nature through
movement, mindful eating, fasting, and fostering connections, we engage
actively in the upward spiral, slowing entropy and optimizing health.

In sum, gravity might be the default setting; entropy and aging happen naturally. Yet grace is intentional. It's the deliberate effort to reverse, rebuild, and
uplift us above the inevitable pull.

Whether it's through fasting to trigger autophagy, meditating to quiet
oxidative stress, or exercising to build strength against gravity's pull, each practice teaches us collaboration with grace and rewrites our biological age and
healthspan, the true art of living well.

My Father: A Life of Legacy

As I reflect on my journey toward understanding the essence of existence, I
am continually drawn back to the figure of my father, an embodiment of many
themes we've explored in this chapter. A civil engineer by profession, he dedicated his life to building public structures, making a tangible impact on the
city of New York. His work included parts of the iconic dinosaur wing at the
American Museum of Natural History, a structure that continues to inspire
awe in countless visitors. His legacy is woven through brick and steel and the

intricate craftsmanship of wood and art he cherished dearly.

My father's hands were gifted. He created small furniture pieces that still hold a place of honor in our home, each one a testament to his commitment to quality and beauty. He taught me that life's creations, whether buildings or furniture, are extensions of ourselves, artifacts that tell our stories long after we're gone.

Until the age of 80, my father thrived without any significant health issues. His memory was sharp, he maintained a vegetable garden that flourished under his attentive care, and his artistic spirit continued to blossom. It wasn't until he developed an aggressive form of lymphoma that his health began to decline. During his hospital stay, all he had was his cell phone, a lifeline to the world outside those sterile walls.

One day, during what would be some of his final moments with me, he showed me a picture of a young sailor and asked if I knew who it was. When I admitted that I didn't, he told me the story behind the portrait, revealing a hidden chapter of his life. The sailor was the son of a distant cousin in India, a woman born with disabilities. After her parents passed away, her family shunned her, leaving her on the brink of homelessness, and forcing her to beg on the streets.

My father extended his hand across continents. He made a promise: "As long as I am alive, you will not need to beg." For years, he quietly followed through on that promise, funding her education and empowering her to find work, ultimately helping her to marry and raise a family of her own. Unbeknownst to us, he had changed their lives forever, eventually paving the way for their son to become a sailor.

As he reflected on this story, his voice was infused with quiet strength and humility. He told me, "Kavin, the greatest gift you have is your ability to give." He posed a question that still echoes in my mind:

"When all others walk out, are you the one who walks in?"

It was a profound insight into the nature of generosity and purpose, illustrating that we can contribute to something that transcends our existence in our finite lives.

When my father passed, I opened his phone, intent on gathering pictures for his memorial. To my surprise, he had only five images saved on his device: a photo of him with my mother, one of me and my family, a picture of my brother and his family, a picture of the sailor, and one of the temple where he worshipped. In those five images lay the essence of his life, the connections that meant everything, the realities he cherished most.

This moment offered me insight into a powerful truth. Ultimately, friends, life boils down to a handful of things that truly give it meaning. I urge you to contemplate this: **If you distill your life down to five pictures that hold true significance, what would they be?** Allow those images to infuse your existence with lasting purpose and connection.

Invest your time and energy in relationships and pursuits that will echo beyond your years. True fulfillment arises from these interactions, fostering a sense of belonging that nourishes the heart and soul and contributes to health and well-being. In the end, like my father, our greatest legacy may reside not in what we achieved during our time but in how we uplifted the lives of those around us.

Hero to Zero

As AI races ahead, transforming the world at breakneck speed, we face a choice: evolve or become obsolete. If we fail to reconnect with our primal intelligence, we'll have hyper-capable technology but a humanity that's utterly incapable of being truly alive.

When we are young, we're all chasing the need for more: wealth, influence, and relationships. I checked off all those boxes. Yet, an unshakable void remained.

Then I stumbled upon *Inner Engineering: A Yogi's Guide to Joy* by Sadhguru, and one line shattered my worldview: **"The less you are, the more life is."** Until then, I had dismissed mindfulness and meditation as spa-day fluff, something you did to take the edge off. But as I dug deeper, I realized their purpose wasn't to dull the mind but to awaken it. It wasn't about stopping thoughts (which, if you've ever tried, is like trying not to picture a pink elephant). It was about moving beyond thought to experience life as it *is*.

That insight pulled me into a deep inward dive. The first step? Taming the monkey mind. Imagine aligning all the iron atoms in a chunk of metal; it turns into a magnet. That's what focus does to the mind. But anyone who's tried meditation knows that the monkey doesn't like sitting still. The real challenge isn't just learning to pay attention, it's evolving that attention into a state of pure awareness.

And here's the paradox: **The more we let go of who we think we are, the more life reveals who we *truly* are.** We're so full of our own identities, that is, our likes, dislikes, and ideologies, that there's no space for something bigger to take root.

But in that spaciousness, something profound emerges: compassion.

There's a light within each of us, buried beneath layers of conditioning, that has the power to illuminate the world. But we stay trapped in the roles we play, the hero of our own story, when in reality, life is far grander than any one of *us*. The moment we stop seeing ourselves as the main character, our experience of life deepens.

When we truly feel connected to all of humanity, no one needs to lecture us on cultural competency; it's built-in. When our awareness expands to an all-inclusive consciousness, the *hero* dissolves into a zero, and suddenly, caring for the planet and each other becomes second nature.

The ultimate upgrade is the shift from a survival mode of scarcity and self-preservation to a life of connection, compassion, and contribution. Each day offers another layer to peel back, another opportunity to let our light shine in a world that needs it now more than ever.

The Infinite in the Finite

As we conclude this chapter, we revisit the paradox that defines our existence:

While our lives are undoubtedly finite, the impact we make, the love we share, and the connections we cultivate have the potential to stretch into infinity. Embracing our mortality is not a cause for despair but a compelling invitation to live more meaningfully, healthfully, and vibrantly. It encourages us to infuse our everyday experiences with purpose and intention, reminding us that every moment is precious, the essence of our true vitality.

As Rumi wisely said, **"Try not to resist the changes that come your way. Instead, let life live through you. And do not worry that your life is turning upside down. How do you know that the side you are used to is better than the one to come?"** Let this perspective guide you as you navigate your journey, transforming the fleeting nature of life into an endless well of inspiration, connection, and love.

So, as you step into the world, embrace the radiant possibilities that await. Live fully, connect deeply, and remember:

By understanding our finite nature, we unlock life's infinite beauty.

Primal Practices:

Within this vast universe, we are not separate. We *are* the cosmos, made of stardust, animated by the same forces that swirl galaxies and birth supernovas.

But in the noise of modern life, we forget this connection. We shrink into deadlines, notifications, and self-imposed urgencies. We lose sight of the grand mystery.

The good news? Reconnecting doesn't require a telescope, a physics degree, or a monk's retreat to the Himalayas. It simply requires *practice*. Here are seven ways to break free from the illusion of smallness and step into your cosmic nature:

1. Breathe Like a Cosmic Traveler

Breath is our first and last act in this life, yet we rush through it as if it's trivial. Slow down. Take five deep, deliberate breaths right now. Feel the oxygen, formed in ancient stars, enter your lungs, fuel your cells, and cycle through your body. Every inhale is a reunion with the universe. Every exhale, a surrender to its rhythm.

2. Worship at the Altar of Nature

Step outside and be with the earth. No agenda. No distractions. Just watch the clouds drift, listen to the wind, or press your hands against the bark of a tree that has been breathing longer than you. The cosmos doesn't only exist in deep space; it pulses in the rivers, forests, and even the soil beneath your feet.

3. Engage with Awe, Daily

Awe is a portal to the infinite. Stare at the stars. Watch a sunrise without glancing at your phone. Listen to music so profoundly moving that it makes time disappear. Read something that bends your perception of reality. Awe shatters the illusion of separateness and places you back in the flow of something grander.

4. Move Like an Animal, Not a Machine

You weren't designed to sit at a desk all day, disconnected from the primal rhythms of motion. Stretch, jump, climb, run barefoot on grass. Move with intention. Feel your body as part of nature, not apart from it. The more in sync you are with your body, the more in sync you are with life itself.

5. Reclaim the Ritual of Reflection

At the end of each day, take 10 minutes to write, think, or simply sit with the question: **What did today teach me?** Reflection is a cosmic practice; it aligns your finite life with a greater unfolding. Some nights, the answer will be profound. On other nights, it will be simple. But every night, you will grow.

6. Live with Cosmic Gratitude

The odds of *you* existing right now are nearly zero. And yet, here you are. Out of infinite possibilities, you were chosen to experience this. Don't let that miracle go unnoticed. Each morning, name three things you're grateful for, small or grand. Gratitude isn't just a mood boost; it's an act of recognizing the cosmic gift of existence.

7. Become the Light That Expands

The sun doesn't shine for itself; it shines because that's what it *is*. You, too, are light. And the more you expand beyond ego, beyond self-imposed limits, the more you illuminate others. Practice compassion, not as an obligation, but as your natural state. Help, share, uplift, not because you *should*, but because you *are* the cosmos in human form.

Final Thought: Remember, You Belong to the Stars

You don't need to escape to the wilderness or study astrophysics to connect with the infinite. You are already woven into it. The universe is not out there; it's within you, around you, through you. Practice these seven simple rituals, and watch your perspective shift from small to vast, from isolated to interconnected.

Live fully. Breathe deeply. Wonder often.

The cosmos is waiting.

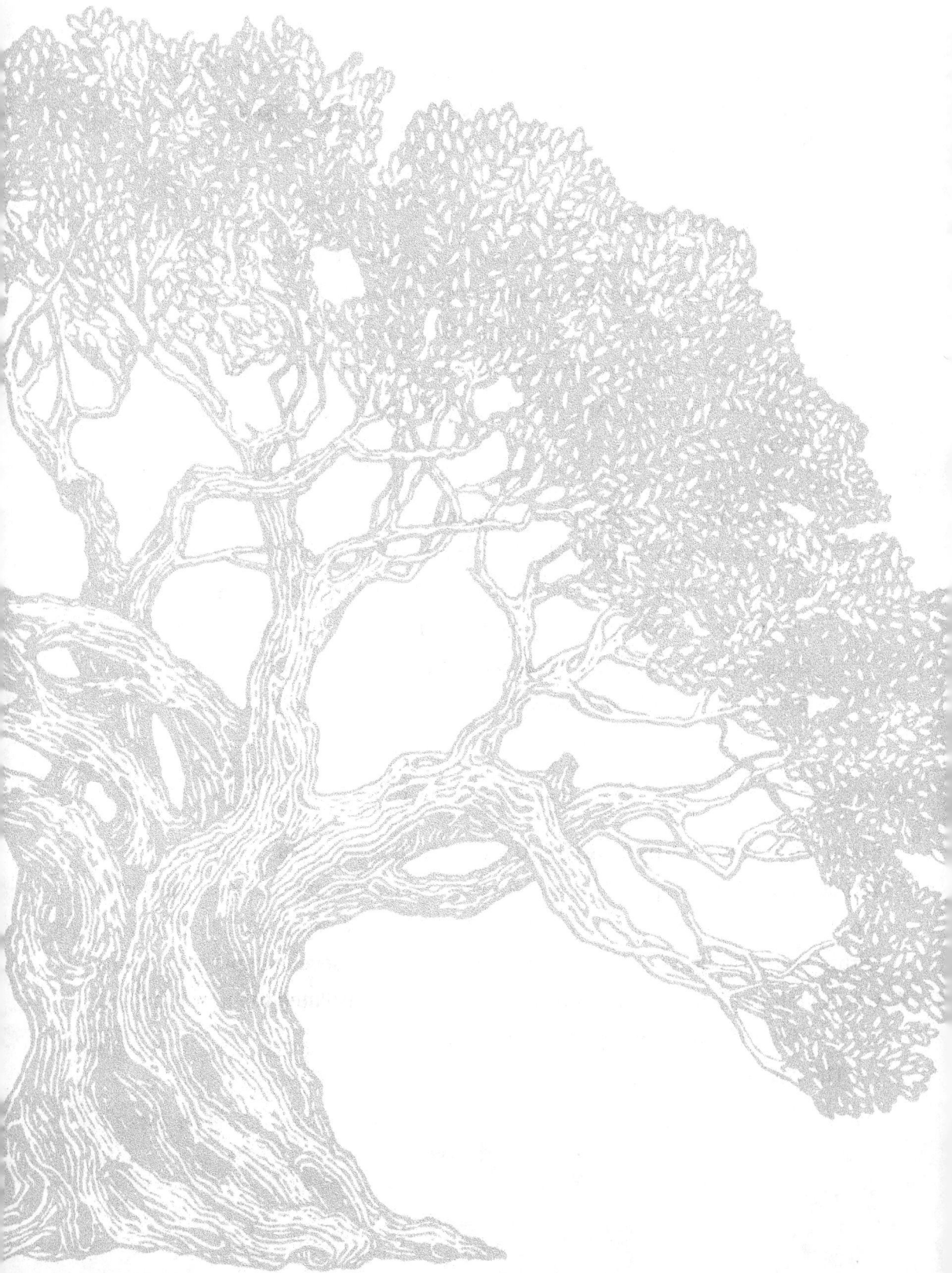

8

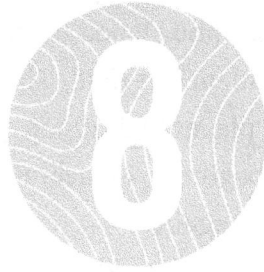

PRIMAL RESET PROGRAM: RETURNING TO OUR NATURAL RHYTHMS

Let go of Old Paradigms

In the whispering dawn of spring, a farmer stands before his fields, seeds of promise in hand. These are no ordinary seeds. They are the blueprints of renewal, the architects of a bountiful harvest. But the soil before him is hardened, depleted from seasons past, unyielding to the gentle touch of new beginnings. He knows, as all seasoned farmers do, that scattering seeds onto this crusted ground would be an exercise in futility. Growth cannot take root in resistance. First, the soil must be broken, turned, and softened; only then can it welcome new life.

This act of tilling is not merely agricultural; it is metaphorical. It is what we must do with our minds before true transformation can begin. The paradigms we hold, the ingrained beliefs about health, aging, and vitality, are like that hardened soil. Many of these beliefs served a purpose once, but now they are relics of an outdated operating system, stifling our ability to evolve. Before installing the **7 Key Paradigms to Reverse Biological Age**, we must examine, challenge, and dismantle old concepts.

Consider the story of the drumming instructor with two students. The first is a blank slate, eager to learn, unburdened by past experiences. The second is an experienced drummer, confident but rigid. The teacher charges the beginner $45 an hour, but the seasoned player $85. When questioned about the price difference, he explains, "For the beginner, I teach. For the experienced one, I must first un-teach before I can teach again."

This is the challenge we face. Our old habits, deeply entrenched, demand unlearning before we can truly adopt new ways of thinking. If we cling to outdated paradigms—that aging is an inevitable decline, that stress is a badge of honor, that exhaustion is proof of productivity—we leave no room for the profound truth: **Health, strength, and vibrancy are within our grasp at any age.** The work begins with breaking the mental ground, making space for something better.

No Pain, No Gain? More Like No Balance, No Gain

The old gym mantra "no pain, no gain" has been parroted for decades, convincing us that suffering is the only path to growth. But what if the real secret to longevity isn't found in pushing harder but in recalibrating to create balance? What if true strength isn't about enduring more pain but cultivating resilience through recovery?

Modern science is rewriting the script on wellness, shifting the focus from overexertion to equilibrium. At the heart of this transformation lies the autonomic nervous system, where the vagus nerve, the maestro of our "rest and digest" functions, plays a crucial role. As we have discussed, high vagal tone has been linked to reduced stress, improved emotional regulation, and lower inflammation. In essence, the body's built-in recovery mechanism counterbalances the stress response many people overindulge in.

Yet, we continue to glorify relentless effort while ignoring the biological imperative for stillness. Meditation, deep breathing, and deliberate recovery aren't indulgences but performance enhancers. They allow the body to thrive instead of merely endure. By shifting from "no pain, no gain" to "stillness prevents illness," we open the door to a more intelligent approach where effort and recovery work in harmony rather than opposition.

True health isn't about burning ourselves out; it's about burning our fire bright without letting it consume us.

The Microbial Misconception: Why a Little Dirt is Good for You

For decades, we've waged war on bacteria, scrubbing, sanitizing, and sterilizing every surface in the name of health. The message has been clear: Cleanliness is next to godliness, and microbes are the enemy. But we may have done more harm than good in our quest for purity.

The truth is, bacteria aren't our adversaries, they're our allies. As we discussed, our gut microbiome, a teeming ecosystem of trillions of microorganisms, plays a crucial role in digestion, immunity, metabolism, and even mental health. Research has linked a diverse microbiome to lower levels of anxiety and depression, reduced inflammation, and improved metabolic function. But our modern obsession with sterility, with antibacterial soaps, excessive antibiotic use, and hyper-sanitized environments, has stripped away the microbial diversity that keeps us resilient.

This war on microbes doesn't just affect our guts. It extends to our entire immune system. The "hygiene hypothesis" suggests that early exposure to bacteria and dirt helps train our immune systems, reducing the risk of allergies, asthma, and autoimmune diseases later in life. Without these early microbial interactions, our immune system behaves like an untrained guard dog, either overreacting to harmless stimuli or failing to respond effectively to real threats.

So, what's the solution? Microbial diplomacy. Instead of eliminating bacteria, we should be nurturing them. Eating fiber-rich and fermented foods, spending time in nature, gardening, and even letting kids play in the dirt all help cultivate a robust microbiome. True health isn't found in a sterilized bubble but in a dynamic relationship with the natural world. The next time you feel the urge to wage microbial war, consider extending a truce, because the allies you need for better health are already inside you, waiting to be cultivated.

The Elusive Perfect Diet

Society treats nutrition like a moving target, constantly shifting from one extreme to the next. One year, it's low-fat; the next, it's low-carb. Veganism battles carnivorism in an endless war of conflicting ideologies. But the truth is simple: **No single diet fits all.**

What works for one person may not work for another, and attempting to force the body into a rigid mold often does more harm than good. Instead of following dietary dogma, we need to honor our biological individuality. A plant-based, whole-food diet has been consistently linked to longevity and disease prevention. Still, flexibility, rather than strict adherence to rules, allows the body to truly thrive.

Rather than treating our plates as battlegrounds, we should see them as canvases that are vibrant, diverse, and reflective of the nourishment we need. The perfect diet isn't found in a rulebook but in finding what fuels us best.

Twist, Bend, Break: The Myth of Fitness

Modern fitness culture has overcomplicated what should be simple. We twist, bend, and contort ourselves into convoluted workouts when the foundation of health has always been built on basic, functional movement.

Squatting, hanging, walking, and lifting are primal movements our bodies evolved to do. Instead of chasing the latest fitness trend, returning to these basics builds true resilience. Research shows that simple, functional movements improve mobility, joint health, and longevity far more effectively than flashy routines designed to look good on social media.

Instead of treating fitness as an aesthetic pursuit, we should reframe it as an investment in our ability to move through life with ease. **The strongest bodies are not the ones sculpted for show, but the ones built for purpose.**

The Brain: A Work in Progress

For decades, the prevailing belief was that the brain's development was largely set in stone by adulthood. This outdated notion painted a grim picture, one where cognitive decline was inevitable, and learning capabilities sharply diminished with age. However, modern neuroscience tells a different story. The concept of neuroplasticity, the brain's continuing ability to form and reorganize synaptic connections, proves that our minds remain dynamic and adaptable throughout life.

Research has shown that even in adulthood, engaging in mentally stimulating activities such as learning a new language, playing a musical instrument, or picking up a new hobby like painting or dancing can significantly reshape the brain. These activities strengthen neural pathways, foster creativity, and delay cognitive decline. Instead of resigning ourselves to mental stagnation, we should embrace continuous learning and exploration, knowing that every challenge we undertake contributes to a healthier, more resilient brain.

The Sleep Paradox: Quality Over Quantity

One of the most widespread sleep myths is that everyone must get precisely eight hours of sleep per night. While adequate rest is undeniably crucial for overall health, the quality of sleep often outweighs the simple number of hours spent in bed.

Studies indicate that deep and REM sleep are essential for memory consolidation, emotional regulation, and overall cognitive function. Maintaining a consistent sleep schedule, keeping bedroom temperatures cool, and reducing exposure to blue light before bed significantly improve sleep efficiency. One well-rested individual may function optimally on six to seven hours of high-quality sleep, while another may require nine. Rather than rigidly trying to achieve an arbitrary number of hours of sleep, optimizing sleep hygiene to enhance overall well-being is more beneficial.

The Metabolism Myth: Age is Not the Enemy

A common misconception suggests that metabolism drastically decreases after a certain age, leading to inevitable weight gain. While it's true that metabolic rates undergo gradual shifts, the change is not as dramatic as many believe. Recent studies indicate that metabolism remains relatively stable from ages 20 to 60, with only minor declines afterward. The real culprits behind midlife weight gain are often decreased physical activity, increased stress levels, and shifts in dietary habits, rather than a significant drop in metabolic function.

Resistance training, regular daily movement, and protein-rich nutrition are key to maintaining a healthy metabolism. Strength training helps preserve lean muscle mass, which is vital in keeping metabolism efficient. Instead of accepting weight gain as an unavoidable part of aging, individuals can take proactive steps to maintain a strong and active body well into later years.

The Cardio Conundrum: More Isn't Always Better

Another long-standing belief is that endless cardio sessions are the best way to lose weight and improve heart health. While cardiovascular exercise is undeniably beneficial, excessive endurance training can lead to diminishing returns and adverse effects, such as increased cortisol levels, muscle loss, and joint stress.

A more balanced approach includes a combination of strength training, high-intensity interval training (HIIT), and moderate aerobic exercise. Strength training enhances metabolic function and bone density, while HIIT provides cardiovascular benefits in a relatively short time. Instead of spending hours on a treadmill, incorporating varied forms of exercise ensures efficiency and sustainability in a long-term fitness regimen.

The Longevity Supplement Trap

The modern wellness industry is flooded with "miracle" supplements promising to extend lifespan, boost immunity, and enhance vitality. While certain nutrients, such as omega-3 fatty acids, vitamin D, and magnesium, play essential roles in overall health, no pill can replace the foundational principles of longevity: proper nutrition, movement, sleep, stress management, and social connection.

Relying solely on supplements while neglecting lifestyle fundamentals is a misguided approach. Whole, nutrient-dense foods provide the body with bioavailable vitamins and minerals in a way that synthetic supplements cannot replicate. Rather than chasing quick fixes, prioritizing a well-balanced diet, physical activity, and emotional well-being is the key to a long and healthy life.

The Hydration Misconception: Do You Need Eight Glasses?

We've all heard it: Drink eight glasses of water daily for optimal health. While hydration is crucial, the "eight-glass rule" is an oversimplification that doesn't account for individual needs, activity levels, climate, or dietary factors. Water intake should be personalized; someone engaging in intense exercise or living in a hot climate naturally requires more fluids than a sedentary person in a cooler environment.

Moreover, hydration comes from various sources, including fruits, vegetables, herbal teas, and even coffee. A more effective strategy is to listen to thirst cues, monitor urine color (light yellow indicates good hydration), and adjust fluid intake based on physical demands rather than adhering to a rigid formula.

Rethinking What We Know

Health, fitness, and longevity are complex, multifaceted topics often clouded by myths and misconceptions. While traditional advice may contain elements of truth, mindlessly following outdated principles can lead to suboptimal results. By embracing science-backed strategies such as continuous learning, prioritizing sleep quality over quantity, engaging in balanced exercise routines, and focusing on holistic health rather than quick fixes, we empower ourselves to lead longer, healthier, and more fulfilling lives.

As we adopt the 7 Key Paradigms, let's return to the farmer's wisdom. His soil, once barren, now tilled, awaits new seeds. No longer rigid with old paradigms, our minds are ready for fresh perspectives.

To break the hardened ground, question what you've been taught about health, aging, and wellness. Challenge the myths that no longer serve you. And then, with open minds and fertile ground, we can plant the seeds of a new way forward, one rooted in strength, intelligence, and vitality.

Constructing Your Life Suspension Bridge

Life moves fast, relentlessly fast. Parents juggle diaper changes, carpool duty, and last-minute school projects. High school and college students drown in exams, deadlines, and the social rollercoaster of young adulthood. Executives operate under the weight of high-stakes meetings and endless to-do lists, often pushing health to the margins. In a world where busyness is both a badge of honor and an unrelenting force, who has time to focus on health and longevity?

The truth is, no one *finds* time. You *make* time. And the secret lies in the natural rhythm of your day, the bookends that hold it all together: your mornings and evenings.

Engineers have long marveled at the power of suspension bridges. Unlike other structures, which rely on numerous support pillars along their span, suspension bridges are held up by just two anchor points, one at each end. Yet, these structures, such as the Golden Gate Bridge or the Brooklyn Bridge, carry immense loads with effortless grace, spanning vast distances without crumbling under their own weight.

Your life is no different. You don't need a complicated, all-day wellness routine. You need strong anchors, AM and PM habits that support the structure of your day. Like the towers of a suspension bridge, these habits provide stability amid the chaos of work, family, and responsibilities. They ensure that you remain balanced, energized, and on course, no matter how turbulent the middle of your day becomes.

Engineering Your Daily Bookends

Most people assume that health requires an all-or-nothing approach: hours at the gym, perfectly portioned organic meals, and a meditation practice so serene it belongs in a Zen monastery. Not true. The key is designing a set of intentional, repeatable habits that integrate seamlessly into the most predictable parts of your day: the beginning and the end. These routines are the foundation of your suspension bridge, ensuring your well-being is preserved even when the middle of your day feels like a hurricane.

So, what do these bookends look like? They don't have to be elaborate. They shouldn't be. They should be simple, powerful, and rooted in the seven key paradigms that reverse biological age and promote lasting vitality.

The AM Ritual: A Strong Takeoff

Mornings set the tone for the day. How we rise determines the energy, focus, and resilience we carry into the hours ahead. In the modern world, the morning often starts with a jolt, maybe an alarm clock or a buzzing phone, and a rush out the door. But what if we instead reclaimed the morning as a primal reset?

At its core, an AM ritual should anchor us in the key elements of primal health: physical, mental, emotional, and existential well-being. This could mean beginning the day with a simple practice that connects us to the earth, such as stepping outside barefoot, breathing in crisp morning air, or feeling sunlight on our skin. It might involve movement intended to engage the body in a way that wakes it up with intention rather than force. It could be a mental or emotional check-in like setting a purposeful direction for the day, engaging in a moment of gratitude, or reconnecting with what truly matters before the world's noise takes over.

Just like a well-built bridge doesn't sway under pressure, a strong AM ritual reinforces our ability to navigate whatever challenges come our way. It's not about rigid routines but designing a morning rhythm that serves as a launchpad for health, clarity, and strength.

The PM Ritual: A Deliberate Landing

If mornings are the takeoff, evenings are the landing. Yet, too often, the modern world robs us of this transition. Work bleeds into home life, screens hijack our attention, and we collapse into bed with an overstimulated brain and an exhausted body. But, like any well-balanced suspension bridge, a day is only as strong as its endpoint.

The PM ritual is an opportunity to realign with our primal health model, to recalibrate the mind-body connection, release the weight of the day, and prepare for deep, restorative sleep. This could be a moment to disconnect from artificial overstimulation and reconnect with something tangible (warm light, soft fabrics, the rhythm of our breath). It might involve an intentional mental shift, for example, letting go of unresolved tension, reflecting on the day's wins, or simply allowing stillness to take over. It might include nourishment, not just through food, but through connection with loved ones, a personal passion, or a deeper existential awareness of our place in an infinite world.

These evening practices don't have to be elaborate, but they must be intentional. They serve as the stabilizing anchor that allows the body to repair, the mind to settle, and the soul to breathe. A strong PM ritual ensures that no matter how chaotic the day has been, we return to the center, ready to rise again tomorrow.

Your Bridge, Your Design

Health is not about rigid discipline or endless lists of to-dos. It's about structure, like a suspension bridge, which isn't held together by excess weight but by strategic tension. The AM and PM rituals serve as the two strongest pillars of our lives, keeping us grounded in what truly matters while allowing us to carry the load of modern demands. By designing these bookends intentionally, we don't just survive the day, we truly live it.

Let us explore each of these domains—physical, mental, emotional, and existential—more deeply, providing tangible ways to integrate them into a strong, sharp, and enduring life. When the anchors are strong, the bridge can hold any weight.

This book isn't about giving you another checklist of wellness trends to follow mindlessly. It's about crafting a strategy that works for you, a system that transforms your mornings and evenings into powerful tools for health and longevity. Like a suspension bridge, your strength doesn't come from what happens in the middle, it comes from the foundation you build at both ends.

So, what do your bookends look like? The choice is yours. But know this: When you intentionally design your mornings and evenings, you are no longer at the mercy of a busy life. You take control. You set the terms. And you build a bridge to a future of vitality, resilience, and strength.

Priming Physical Health

In the grand architecture of life, physical health is the bedrock, the foundation upon which everything else is built. Without it, our ambitions, creativity, and even our purpose become castles on shifting sand. No matter how brilliant your mind or how noble your mission, if your body falters, everything else is in jeopardy.

The healthier the body, the sharper the mind. Yet modern life has pulled us so far from this primal truth that we often treat our bodies like afterthoughts, machines to be pushed, punished, and occasionally repaired. But our ancestors understood better. Health was not an afterthought; it was the foundation of existence.

In the Primal Health Design model, physical health rests on three pillars: **connection with the earth, connection with the body, and connection with food.** These are not fads or biohacks. They are deep-rooted biological imperatives, core programming written into our DNA long before we were drowning in emails, processed foods, and artificial lighting.

The Forgotten Art of Waking with the Earth

In the chapter on *Grounded Greatness*, we explored many ways to reconnect with the earth: walking barefoot, touching the soil, and immersing ourselves in nature. But there is one primal connection so deeply embedded in our biology that we rarely think about it: **our circadian rhythm.**

Our bodies are not meant to function on artificial schedules dictated by alarm clocks, blue-light screens, and caffeine-fueled mornings. At our core, we are creatures of the earth, designed to wake with the sun's rising and rest as it sets. This rhythm, encoded in every cell, governs our sleep, hormones, metabolism, and mental clarity. When we live in sync with this rhythm, we thrive. When we fight it, we deteriorate.

Brahma Murat: The Creator's Hour

In Indian tradition, there is a sacred window of time known as **Brahma Murat,** or the "Creator's Hour." This period, roughly **90 minutes before sunrise,** is revered as the most auspicious time of day. It is the quietest, purest, most potent time for clarity and intention-setting. The name itself holds meaning: *Brahma,* the Creator, and *Murat,* time. This is when creation is most active, not just in the spiritual sense, but biologically.

Yogic literature suggests that when the body is properly aligned with the earth's rhythms, it will naturally wake up during this time. Long before alarm clocks, before schedules dictated by fluorescent-lit offices, our ancestors rose with the shift of the earth's energy. The Hadzabe, the tribal people near whom I spent my childhood in Africa, naturally rose in the early morning, long before the sun was up. They didn't set alarms or check their sleep cycles; they simply *woke,* not out of obligation, but because their bodies responded to the earth itself.

Today, most people do the opposite. Instead of waking with intention, they wake in reaction, hitting snooze, scrambling into the day, chasing a schedule that is already running ahead of them. But Brahma Murat offers an alternative: Instead of waking to the *world's* demands, you wake for *yourself.* You create your day rather than getting dragged into it.

To wake for Brahma Murat, you must first plan for it. And here's where most people get it wrong: waking up early isn't about the morning, it's about the *night before.* If you're scrolling your phone at midnight, your body won't care how spiritual 4:30 a.m. is. If you don't prioritize sleep, you'll be fighting biology, not working with it.

This means setting an **alarm for bedtime, not just for waking up.** It means honoring the natural wind-down cycle, dimming artificial light, and respecting sleep as non-negotiable. Because here's the irony: Early risers aren't "disciplined." They're simply in rhythm with their biology. They don't *force* themselves up; they *align* themselves with the earth's cycles.

The natural world stirs before sunrise. The trees begin their slow exchange of oxygen. Birds begin their first songs. The air itself shifts. This is the **earth's awakening**; we are meant to rise with it.

The modern world has disconnected us from this primal rhythm, but the connection is still there, waiting to be reclaimed. Wake before the world does.

Step outside. Feel the quiet, the stillness, the energy of creation itself. *This* is when clarity comes. *This* is when purpose sharpens.

When you master this rhythm, life stops feeling like something you react to and becomes something you create.

Reconnect with the Earth

Reconnecting with the earth is not a grand, once-in-a-while event; it's a daily practice, a rhythm to be cultivated. Much like a well-carved piece of wood, the body takes shape through repeated, intentional movements. In my lineage of woodworking, the finest pieces aren't forced into form; they are revealed through consistent, mindful refinement. The same applies to our health. The more we shape our lives around the natural world, the more we return to the blueprint nature intended for us.

☼ Morning Rituals: Rise, Align, Energize

GROUNDING: Recharging Your Bioelectrical Circuit

Your body is an electrical system, and like any system, it needs stable ground. The Hadzabe didn't need studies to tell them this. They simply *lived* it, barefoot, in constant contact with the earth. Living indoors in the modern world, by contrast, insulates us from this vital connection.

HOW TO DO IT:

Step outside **barefoot** on grass, soil, or sand for at least **5 to 10 minutes** in the morning. This practice, grounding, allows you to absorb the earth's free electrons, which may help lower inflammation, stabilize cortisol, and improve sleep quality. If you live in a city, consider conductive wearing shoes outdoors; they mimic the effect of walking barefoot.

MORNING SUN: The Master Reset for Your Body Clock

Light profoundly impacts brain function. Morning sunlight isn't just about vitamin D, it's about **resetting your circadian rhythm, optimizing mitochondrial function, and regulating mood and energy.** In India, this wisdom has been practiced for millennia. When you expose your eyes and skin to the morning sun, you're aligning yourself with this innate rhythm.

HOW TO DO IT:

> Within **30 minutes of waking,** step outside for **15-20 minutes of direct sunlight.** No sunglasses. No windows filtering the light. Bonus points if you combine this with a morning barefoot walk or stretching session.

COLD EXPOSURE: Cultivate Your Thermoregulation

Our ancestors didn't have thermostats. They adapted to the elements, and in doing so, they built resilience. Modern life, with its climate control and thermal insulation, has made us **fragile**. Cold exposure activates **brown fat, sharpens the nervous system, and strengthens immunity.**

HOW TO DO IT:

> • Start with **30 seconds of cold water** at the end of your shower. Gradually increase over time.
>
> • If you're ready for the deep plunge, try **ice baths** (50°F for 2-5 minutes).
>
> • In winter, **ditch excessive layers of clothing** for short, controlled exposure to the cold. Let

your body *remember* what it means to generate its own heat.

NATURE IMMERSION: Bathing in Biodiversity

The Japanese call it *Shinrin Yoku*, or **forest bathing**. The Hadzabe didn't have a name for it; it was simply *life*. When you immerse yourself in nature, your body absorbs unseen benefits: **negative ions from waterfalls, microbiome diversity from soil, phytoncides from trees**, all working silently to regulate your stress response, boost your immunity, and enhance cognitive function.

HOW TO DO IT:

- Walk in a **forest, park, or near a waterfall** at least **once a week.**

- **Touch the earth**—sit, breathe, and let the environment recalibrate your nervous system.

- For urban dwellers, use air purifiers or ionizers to bring some of these benefits into your home.

☾ Evening Rituals: Unwind, Restore, Sync with the Earth

GARDENING GRATITUDE: Microbiome Medicine

Soil isn't just dirt; it's **medicine for your gut and immune system**. Every handful contains **millions of microorganisms** that communicate with your microbiome, strengthening your body from the inside out. Studies show that exposure to soil bacteria like *Mycobacterium vaccae* can even act as a natural antidepressant.

HOW TO DO IT:

- **Get your hands in the dirt.** Garden, plant, or even re-pot an indoor plant.

- No yard? Visit a **community garden** or **buy unwashed organic produce** and handle it before you wash off the soil.

BALANCE WALKS: Strengthening Your Foundation

As a radiologist, I see how modern sedentary living **erodes our physical foundation**. Feet are meant to sense, adapt, and stabilize, yet we trap them in rigid shoes and flat surfaces. This dulls our proprioception, the body's ability to sense itself in space, leading to weaker muscles and poor balance.

HOW TO DO IT:

- Walk **barefoot on uneven terrain**, such as grass, sand, or rocks.

- Incorporate **heel-to-toe walking, backward walking, or navigating cobblestones** to engage stabilizing muscles.

CONTRAST THERAPY: The Ancient Recovery Hack

Saunas followed by cold plunges weren't just a Scandinavian tradition; they existed across cultures. This alternating exposure to heat and cold improves **circulation, detoxification, and metabolic health.**

HOW TO DO IT:

- **Cycle between hot and cold**: sauna to cold plunge, hot shower to cold rinse.

- If you can't access a sauna, **switch between hot and cold showers** at night.

Reclaiming the Primal Connection with the Body

Our bodies are ancient instruments designed for movement, adaptability, and resilience. Yet, modern life has shackled them; they are slouched over screens, sedentary for hours, and dulled by artificial comfort. To reconnect with our bodies' primal intelligence, we must honor the daily rituals that align with our evolutionary blueprint.

☀ Morning Rituals: Awaken the Body's Intelligence

Posture Check & Neck Reset
Before stepping out of bed, perform a **chin tuck** (put your index finger on your chin and push your head back) to reset your spinal alignment. Visualize a thread pulling the crown of your head skyward, elongating your spine, and counteracting the tech-induced forward head posture. Stand tall; command the day with confidence.

Functional Wake-Up Call
Instead of rolling out of bed like a crumpled piece of paper, begin with **squatting**, an ancestral movement we've abandoned. Drop into a deep squat for 30 seconds, letting your hips open and your ankles mobilize. Feel stiff? That's your body whispering: *You've forgotten me.*

Hanging: The Primal Shoulder Reset

Find a sturdy pull-up bar or tree branch and hang for 30-60 seconds. This decompresses your spine, strengthens your grip, and restores shoulder health. The Hadza do this naturally. Modern humans? Not so much. Start with bent arms or chair support if a full dead hang is too much.

Proprioception & Barefoot Balance

Stand on one leg while brushing your teeth. This simple act fires up stabilizing muscles, reconnecting you to your primal ability to balance. For an extra challenge, close your eyes to force your nervous system to adapt and refine its awareness of space.

Rucking: The Forgotten Superpower

Strap on a backpack with 15-25 pounds and take a **10-minute brisk morning walk**. This is ancestral fitness in action; weighted walking stimulates bones, muscles, and cardiovascular function without the grind of high-impact exercise. Remember, slow, deliberate movement is just as powerful as HIIT.

☀ Midday Movement: Break the Chains of Sedentarism

Digital Detox & Gaze Elevation

Set an hourly reminder to lift your head and look beyond a screen. Walk to a window, focus on the horizon, and stretch your neck gently. This micro-movement counters hours of downward gazing.

The Squat Break

Instead of sitting on a chair, drop into a resting squat for 30 seconds. Eating, waiting, and thinking can be done in a squat. It's a full-body tune-up hidden in plain sight.

☾ Evening Rituals: Unwind, Recover, & Realign

Tai Chi & Breathwork

Engage in **5 minutes of Tai Chi** or mindful movement before dinner. This stimulates **interoception**, your body's internal awareness, calming the nervous system and enhancing digestion.

Myofascial Release & Foam Rolling

Your muscles accumulate tension throughout the day. Use a **foam roller** or lacrosse ball to release knots. Think of it as ironing out the creases in your body's fabric.

Neck Strengthening & Chin Tucks

Before bed, counteract daily screen strain with **isometric neck exercises**. Press your head gently against your palm in four directions: front, back, left, and right. Finish with 10 slow chin tucks to reinforce alignment.

Stretch & Decompress

End the day with a **spinal decompression stretch**. Lie on your back, knees bent, and let gravity realign your spine. Breathe deeply, signaling to your body that it's time to restore.

Reawakening Our Connection with Food

Somewhere along the way, eating became mechanical, a mindless act performed between emails, meetings, and doom-scrolling through our phones. But food was never meant to be just fuel. It's information, medicine, and connection, a sacred bridge between us and the earth. I learned this early on, growing up in a lineage of woodworkers, where every meal was treated with the same care and craftsmanship as a finely carved masterpiece. Later, my time with the Hadza tribe reinforced this. Food wasn't just sustenance; it was a ritual, a communion with nature.

To reclaim this lost art, we must return to the fundamentals. These daily rituals are designed to transform one's relationship with food, making every meal a moment of intention, nourishment, and vitality.

☀ Morning Rituals: Awaken the Senses

Ease into Intermittent Fasting:

Before reaching for breakfast, pause. Let your body ride the natural metabolic wave of the night a little longer. Start by extending your fasting window gradually, first 12 hours, then 14, eventually reaching 16. During this time, sip warm water, herbal teas, or black coffee to gently support digestion and cellular renewal. Think of it as giving your body time to reset before the day's demands begin.

Mindful Movement on an Empty Stomach :

The Hadzabe don't wake up to a bowl of cereal. They start their day moving by walking, stretching, even sprinting to track prey. You don't need to hunt your breakfast, but a light morning walk, yoga, or stretching while maintaining your nighttime fast helps tap into stored energy, optimizing fat metabolism and mental clarity.

☀ ☾ Midday & Evening Practices: Eating with Intention

Eat with the Seasons and Support the Soil:

Nature has a rhythm, and our diets should reflect it. Prioritize local and seasonal foods. Visit a farmers' market, join a CSA (community-supported agriculture) group, or grow your herbs. When you eat seasonally, you align with nature's wisdom. Plus, supporting regenerative agriculture is one of the most impactful ways to heal your gut microbiome and the planet.

Color Your Plate Like a Painter's Palette:

My woodworking ancestors knew the importance of variety and used different woods for different strengths. Your body thrives the same way. A plate rich in colors, such as deep greens, fiery oranges, and vibrant purples, ensures a broad spectrum of antioxidants, vitamins, and minerals. Make every meal a masterpiece.

Support Gut Resilience with Ferment Foods:

Your gut is home to trillions of microbes that influence everything from digestion to mood. Fermented foods like kimchi, sauerkraut, and kefir introduce beneficial bacteria, allowing your microbiome to function like a well-tuned orchestra. Make it a habit to include a small portion with at least one meal a day.

Master the Art of Mindful Eating:

Put the phone down. Turn off the TV. Chew slowly. Savor each bite like it's the last meal you'll ever have. When you eat mindfully, your brain registers satiety more efficiently, digestion improves, and you forge a deeper appreciation for your food.

Food as Medicine

Prioritize Healthy Fats & Antioxidants:

Your brain is nearly 60% fat. Feed it well. Avocados, wild-caught fish, nuts, and extra virgin olive oil provide essential omega-3s and monounsaturated fats, crucial for cognitive and cardiovascular health. Pair these with antioxidant-rich foods like berries and dark leafy greens to combat inflammation at a cellular level.

Ditch the Processed, Embrace the Whole:

If it comes in a package with a long ingredient list, it's probably better left on the shelf. Whole foods, those close to their natural state, nourish your body in a way that synthetic, ultra-processed alternatives never can.

Stay Curious About Where Your Food Comes From:

Develop a relationship with your food. Visit a farm, learn about soil health, or grow something yourself, even if it's just a pot of basil on your windowsill. When you connect with the origins of your food, you deepen your respect for it nourishing yourself on a different level.

Reclaiming our Mental Health
Mind–Body Connection

We live in a world that demands our attention at every turn. Emails arrive before breakfast, notifications come mid-conversation, and the hum of obligation is ever present. But the body has a rhythm older than time itself, a language of stillness, breath, and movement encoded in our DNA. Mastering the mind-body connection is not about control but deep listening, learning to hear what has always been there.

As a neuroradiologist, I've seen the human brain in ways most never will. I've seen its exquisite design, infinite adaptability, and vulnerability to modern chaos. As someone of Indian origin, I was raised with traditions steeped in mindfulness, breathwork, and yogic wisdom.

Stillness is not the absence of movement, it's the mastery of attention. In a world that thrives on distraction, cultivating stillness is a radical act of self-mastery.

Pick **one or two** of these rituals today. Observe the difference. Over time, you'll feel increased clarity, reduced stress, and a deeper sense of presence. This is not about escaping the world but building an inner world so strong that external chaos no longer controls you.

Be still. Be deliberate. Be primal.

☼ Morning Rituals: Setting the Mental Operating System

The 30-Minute Rule: No External Inputs

When you wake up, your brain is in a highly programmable theta state. Reach for your phone, and you're letting the world's demands program your mind before you take a conscious breath. Instead, spend the first 30 minutes tech-free. Drink water, stretch, sit in silence, go outside for a walk in the sun. This single act resets your dopamine sensitivity, stabilizes cortisol, and prevents the mental chaos of a reactionary day.

Breathwork for Cognitive Priming

Your breath is the remote control for your nervous system. Done right, it's also the fastest way to sharpen your focus. Try this simple **6:6:6:6 box breathing** protocol:

- Inhale for **6 seconds.**

- Hold for **6 seconds.**

- Exhale for **6 seconds.**

- Hold empty for **6 seconds.** Repeat for 5 to 10 minutes. This increases oxygen efficiency, enhances neuroplasticity, and kickstarts a calm yet alert state of mind.

For a more dynamic morning, practice **Kumbhaka (breath retention)**, a technique yogis and elite freedivers use. Inhale deeply, hold until you feel slight discomfort, then exhale fully. This strengthens CO_2 tolerance, improves mitochondrial efficiency, and upgrades brain endurance.

The 4-Second Rule: Pause Before Reacting

Most people live in reflex mode, reacting, replying, making split-second decisions without space to think. **Reclaim that space.** Before responding to anything, be it a text, a conversation, a stressful thought, pause for **four seconds**. Inhale. Hold. Exhale. Then act. This simple habit rewires your brain for higher reasoning and reduces impulsivity.

☾ Evening Rituals: The Primal Sleep Reset

The 90-Minute Digital Wind-Down

Screens after sunset trick your brain into thinking it's still daytime. The result? Melatonin suppression, fragmented sleep, and morning grogginess. The fix is simple:

- 90 minutes before bed, ditch all blue-light screens.

- Use red lights, candles, or dim, warm lighting instead.

- If you must use a screen, wear blue-light-blocking glasses.

The Art of Breathing: Anapanasati Practice

Before bed, spend **5 to 10 minutes** on mindful breathing. Sit comfortably, eyes closed, and focus purely on your breath with no force, just observation. This simple act thickens the prefrontal cortex, reducing anxiety and enhancing mental clarity.

For a deeper dive, try **alternate nostril breathing (Nadi Shodhana):**

- Inhale through the left nostril, closing the right.

- Exhale through the right nostril, closing the left.

- Reverse and repeat for 5 minutes. This activates the parasympathetic nervous system, lowering cortisol and preparing the body for deep sleep.

Core Cooling: A Hunter-Gatherer Sleep Hack

Your ancestors didn't sleep in 72°F climate-controlled bedrooms. They slept in the cold. Why? Because dropping core body temperature is a biological sleep trigger.

- Set your bedroom temp to 65–67°F.

- Take a cold shower or soak your feet in cool water before bed.

- Sleep in light clothing or under a weighted blanket for deeper rest.

Consistency: Aligning with Nature's Clock

Your body craves rhythm. Aim to **wake up and sleep within the same 30-minute window every day**, even on weekends. This will stabilize hormone cycles, boost energy, and increase longevity.

The Mental Offload: Clearing Cognitive Clutter

If your mind races at night, try a **brain dump journal**. Write down unfinished tasks, random thoughts, or emotions, then close the notebook. Your brain interprets this as "handled," reducing subconscious stress. Sleep is not just physical rest; it's psychological processing. Give your brain permission to shut down.

Engaging Emotional Health
Awakening Purpose, Flow, and Ikigai

In our modern world, purpose is often treated like some grand cosmic secret waiting to be found, like an ancient relic buried beneath the sands of time. But here's the truth: Purpose isn't discovered; it's cultivated. Just as a tree doesn't sit around wondering whether it should grow, we are biologically wired for meaning. Neuroscience, evolutionary biology, and ancestral wisdom confirm that purpose is not some esoteric luxury; it's an essential force for well-being, as fundamental to survival as food, movement, and connection.

Purpose strengthens neural pathways, shapes cognition, and fuels motivation. Growing up with the Hadzabe, I witnessed people whose purpose was woven seamlessly into daily life as they hunted, gathered food, and told stories. They didn't chase purpose; they lived it. Similarly, my woodworking ancestors didn't sit around waiting for inspiration to strike; they shaped their world with their hands.

We don't stumble upon purpose like an explorer discovering a lost city. We *build* it through action, attention, and alignment. Purpose is not something we passively wait for; it's something we cultivate daily through small but deliberate choices. By engaging in these primal practices, you're not just living, you're thriving in sync with the very design of your biology.

Find your flow, ignite your Ikigai, and let your purpose evolve through the life you create every day.

☀ Morning Rituals: Ignite Your Day with Purpose

Set Your Intentions Before Your Feet Hit the Floor

Before your mind gets hijacked by emails and notifications, take a moment. Breathe. Ask yourself, *What's one thing I want to create, impact, or contribute today?* Neuroscientifically speaking, this isn't just wishful thinking, it's priming your brain's reticular activating system (RAS) to filter the world through a lens of purpose.

Deep Work: The Neuroscience of Focus

Multitasking is a myth. Purpose thrives in the realm of deep *work*, uninterrupted, immersive engagement. Studies show that focused work strengthens myelin production, enhancing cognitive function. Whether writing, sculpting, designing, or solving complex problems, carve out sacred time for uninterrupted flow.

Engage in a Craft—Use Your Hands

Hands-on work is not just therapeutic; it's ancestral. Whether it's woodworking, painting, gardening, or even cooking, tactile engagement activates the sensorimotor cortex, creating a neural feedback loop that enhances patience, problem-solving, and fulfillment. My ancestors shaped wood into art; I shape ideas into understanding. Both fuel purposes.

Trace the Origins of Your Fascination

What did you obsess over as a child? What makes hours feel like minutes? Evolutionarily speaking, your childhood curiosities hold clues to your innate strengths and purpose. Follow them.

☾ Evening Rituals: Ground, Reflect, and Strengthen Your Purpose

Engage in Flow Activities

Flow, the state of being completely absorbed in an activity, is where purpose thrives. Whether it's music, writing, hiking, or problem-solving, intentionally engage in something that makes you lose track of time. Studies show that regular flow experiences enhance dopamine production, reinforcing a sense of fulfillment and motivation.

Reflect on Your Skills

Before bed, take five minutes to jot down three things you did well today. Recognizing your strengths rewires your brain for confidence and reinforces purpose. Over time, this simple habit cultivates an unshakable sense of self-efficacy.

Tell Your Story—Make Sense of Your Journey

The human brain is wired for narrative. Studies on memory and cognition reveal that people who frame their life experiences within a coherent story experience less anxiety and greater clarity. Journaling, reflecting, and sharing your journey isn't just therapy, it's biology. Your life is a story in motion; take an active role in writing it.

Strengthening Bonds with Community and Cause

In the modern world, we've been sold the myth of self-sufficiency—the lone warrior, the independent achiever, the solo success story. But biology tells a different tale. The human brain is wired for connection, and the strongest, longest-living people on the planet aren't those who grind on in isolation, they're those who build and nurture their tribe. Community isn't just a social nicety; it's a survival mechanism, a longevity hack, and a deep wellspring of meaning.

We don't need to abandon modern life to rebuild our tribal instincts. We just need to be intentional. Share meals. Move together. Serve something bigger than yourself. Choose interdependence over isolation. Because at the end of the day, it won't be your to-do list or your productivity that define your life, it will be the strength of your connections.

Morning Rituals: Setting the Foundation for Connection

Start with Gratitude for Your Tribe

Before the day's demands pull you in different directions, take a moment to acknowledge the people in your life. Maybe it's a mental list, a journal entry, or a quick text to someone who matters. Neuroscience confirms that gratitude rewires the brain, strengthening social bonds and increasing happiness. A simple "thinking of you" can ripple outward in ways you can't predict.

Move with Your People

The Hadza don't go to the gym; they walk, hunt, and gather in groups. We thrive when we move together. Instead of a solo workout, try a morning walk with a friend, a group run, or a virtual check-in with an accountability partner. Physical movement in sync with others deepens connection, a phenomenon rooted in our mirror neuron system.

Share a Morning Ritual with Family

Tea with your spouse. A joke with your kids over breakfast. A handshake, a hug, a small moment of presence. The Indian tradition of early-morning chai circles reflects daily connection without distractions. These rituals aren't just habits but the glue that holds relationships together.

☾ Evening Rituals: Closing the Day with Connection

Break Bread—With Presence

Dinner isn't just about eating, it's about anchoring relationships. Whether it's a home-cooked meal or takeout at the table, make a habit of eating with others without screens. The cultures with the longest lifespans in the world all share one thing: meals are communal, unhurried, and filled with conversation.

Build Your Moai—Your Circle for Life

Okinawans call it a Moai, a group of lifelong friends who commit to supporting each other. Who's in yours? Evenings are a great time for connection. Call a friend, check in on family, or set up a weekly gathering. Social resilience is as important as physical health.

Engage in a Ritual of Service

Nothing binds a tribe together like a shared purpose. The best way to strengthen relationships is to serve together. Dedicate an evening once a week to volunteering, mentoring, or contributing to a cause larger than yourself.

Tell the Stories That Matter

We process life through stories. Before bed, instead of scrolling mindlessly, share a meaningful story, such as an experience from your day, a lesson learned, or a memory from your heritage. Neuroscientific research shows that storytelling enhances emotional bonding and strengthens neural pathways of empathy.

Honor the Power of Touch and Eye Contact

A hug. A hand on the shoulder. A look that says, "I see you."

Human connection isn't just words, it's physical, primal, essential. The Hadza touch each other constantly. Before sleep, take a moment to connect physically with those closest to you.

Exploring Existential Health
Connect to Our Finite Life within an Infinite Cosmos

We spend our days as if time is infinite, yet our existence is a flicker in the vast expanse of the cosmos. To truly live, we must first embrace the certainty of our mortality, not as a source of fear but as a compass for meaning. These daily rituals are about clarity. They remind us that each sunrise is a gift, each breath a fleeting miracle, and each moment an invitation to live purposefully. By aligning with the finite and the infinite, we step beyond mere existence into deep, awakened living.

In the modern rush, we often forget a truth: **We are not separate from the universe. We are the universe.** The same elements that forged supernovas flow through our veins. The same rhythms that shape galaxies beat within our hearts. And yet, we spend our days drowning in emails and traffic jams, and scrolling through screens as if we are small and inconsequential.

You don't need a telescope or a spiritual retreat to align with the infinite. The cosmos isn't out there; it's within, around, and through you. Live fully. Breathe deeply. Wonder often.

The universe is waiting.

☀ Morning Rituals: Embracing Mortality with Awareness

Memento Mori Meditation:
Start your day by contemplating the impermanence of life. Reflect on the fact that today is a gift and that awareness should guide your actions, choices, and priorities. This will clarify and sharpen your focus on what truly matters.

Daily Legacy Check-In:
Before diving into the day's tasks, ask yourself: *If today were my last, what would I do differently?* Align your actions with what you want to leave behind.

☾ Evening Rituals: Surrendering to the Infinite

Journal: The Final Page Exercise:
Before bed, write as if today was your last entry in the book of your life. Modern life convinces us that days are for doing and nights are for numbing out. But the wisest traditions, whether in Indian philosophy, African storytelling, or the meditations of great thinkers, know that the day isn't complete until we extract its meaning. Sit with the question: **What did today teach me?** Some nights, the answer will be grand. On other nights, it will be as simple as "take more deep breaths." But in the asking, we align with something timeless.

Engage with Awe Daily
Your brain is wired for wonder. Let it fire. Step outside and look up—yes, really look—at the stars. If you can't see them, watch the movement of the clouds. Listen to music that expands you, read something that bends your perception. Neuroscience tells us that awe recalibrates the brain, shrinking stress and expanding our sense of time. In the Hadza way, awe isn't an event, it's a practice. Make it one of yours.

Sleep with Cosmic Gratitude
The odds of you existing right now are nearly zero. And yet, here you are, a cosmic accident, a miracle of probability, a fleeting yet infinite moment in the grand sweep of time. Before closing

your eyes, name three things you're grateful for. Small or vast, it doesn't matter. This isn't a gimmick; it's a recalibration of your perspective. And perspective is everything.

Throughout the Day: Mortality as a Guide for Deeper Living

Wear a Symbol of Impermanence:
Whether it's a bracelet, a ring, or a simple piece of wood you keep in your pocket, let it serve as a tactile reminder that everything, including you, will one day return to the earth.

Speak as if It's the Last Time:
When talking to loved ones, practice the mindset that this could be your last conversation. It cultivates deeper presence, kindness, and appreciation in every interaction.

Let Nature Teach You:
Observe a leaf falling, a river flowing, or an animal moving effortlessly with life's rhythm. Nature doesn't resist impermanence, it embodies it. Learn from that acceptance.

The Primal Reset: Reclaiming the Intelligence of Your Body

Aging is not the slow ticking of a clock; it's the accumulation of disconnection. Disconnection from movement, from light, from deep rest, from the very forces that built us. And yet, your biology has not forgotten. Your mitochondria, tiny powerhouses in each cell, still remember when humans rose with the sun, moved with purpose, and honored the rhythms of the earth. The *Primal Reset*

Program is not about adding complexity to your life; it's about subtracting the noise and returning to what's essential.

I've spent my career studying the brain, peering into the neural landscapes of thousands of people. I can tell you this: The mind is plastic, the body is adaptive, and decline is *not* inevitable. With the right inputs, you can reshape your biology, rewire your habits, and reverse the markers of aging at the cellular level. It begins with anchoring yourself in the seven key paradigms: Earth, Body, Food, Mind, Purpose, Community, and Finite within the Infinite. These are not abstract principles; they are the scaffolding of health itself.

The Rituals That Reshape You

Your daily rituals are the chisels that sculpt your longevity. In my lineage of woodworking, I learned that a master craftsman doesn't rush the process; he respects the grain of the wood and works with it, not against it. Your biology is no different. When you design your morning and evening routines through the lens of *Primal Health Design*, you align with your body's natural intelligence instead of fighting against it.

Each ritual is a signal to your system, a gentle nudge to either repair or decay. Walk barefoot on the earth and you lower inflammation. Practice deep nasal breathing, activating the parasympathetic nervous system and reducing stress hormones. Eat whole, nutrient-dense foods, and your gut microbiome flourishes, influencing everything from cognition to immunity. Sleep in darkness, and your brain flushes out metabolic waste, sharpening your thinking. These are not trends; they are biological imperatives.

Reversing Biological Age: The Science of Reset

As you integrate these daily practices, you don't just *feel* better, you *become* better at the molecular level. The Primal Reset Program influences key drivers of biological age:

> 1. **Cellular Health:** Your mitochondria power every function in your body. When they thrive, you thrive. Movement, fasting,

and cold exposure stimulate mitochondrial biogenesis, making you more resilient.

2. **Systemic Inflammation:** Chronic inflammation is the silent saboteur behind aging and disease. Grounding, fasting, and consuming polyphenol-rich foods act as natural anti-inflammatories.

3. **Metabolic Health:** Insulin resistance is a modern plague. Training your body to switch between glucose and fat as fuel sources enhances metabolic flexibility, keeping you sharp and energized.

4. **Oxidative Stress:** Antioxidant-rich foods, breathwork, and time in nature mitigate oxidative stress, slowing cellular aging.

5. **Hormonal Balance:** Hormones, from testosterone to estrogen, dictate everything from muscle mass to mood. Sleep, sun exposure, and resistance training are potent hormonal regulators.

6. **Gut Microbiome Diversity:** Your gut is your second brain, influencing immune function, mood, and cognition; fermented foods, fiber, and contact with soil support microbiome diversity.

7. **Functional Age:** Strength, endurance, and agility are better predictors of longevity than your birth certificate. Sprint, lift, move. Your body is designed for it.

8. **Epigenetic Flexibility:** Your genes are not your destiny. They

respond to your lifestyle. Every meal, every workout, every night of deep sleep is an epigenetic signal.

9. **Cognitive Reserve**: Learning, social connection, and meditation build cognitive resilience, delaying neurodegeneration.

10. **Immunosenescence**: Your immune system ages with you but doesn't have to decline. Cold therapy, fasting, and nutrient-dense eating keep it strong.

The Return to a Primal Life

This is not about perfection. It's about alignment. The Hadzabe tribe, who shaped my early understanding of health, don't count calories or track macros, yet they are lean, strong, and metabolically healthy well into old age. Why? Because they live *in rhythm* with the natural world. They move daily, eat whole foods, rest deeply, and connect with their community. They understand something modern life has forgotten: **Longevity is not a product of science alone; it's a result of how we live.**

So, here's the challenge: For 21 days, commit to the *Primal Reset Program*. Strip away the artificial, the over-processed, the over-stimulated. Walk outside at sunrise. Eat real food. Train hard. Breathe deep. Sleep in darkness. Connect with something bigger than yourself. Watch what happens when you stop working against your biology and start working *with* it.

The body is not a machine in need of repair; it is a masterpiece waiting to be restored. You are not meant to wither. You are meant to *thrive*.

Visit PrimalResetProgram.com for a deeper dive and guided instruction on crafting your personalized *Primal Reset Program*. Let's reconnect with our primal lives.

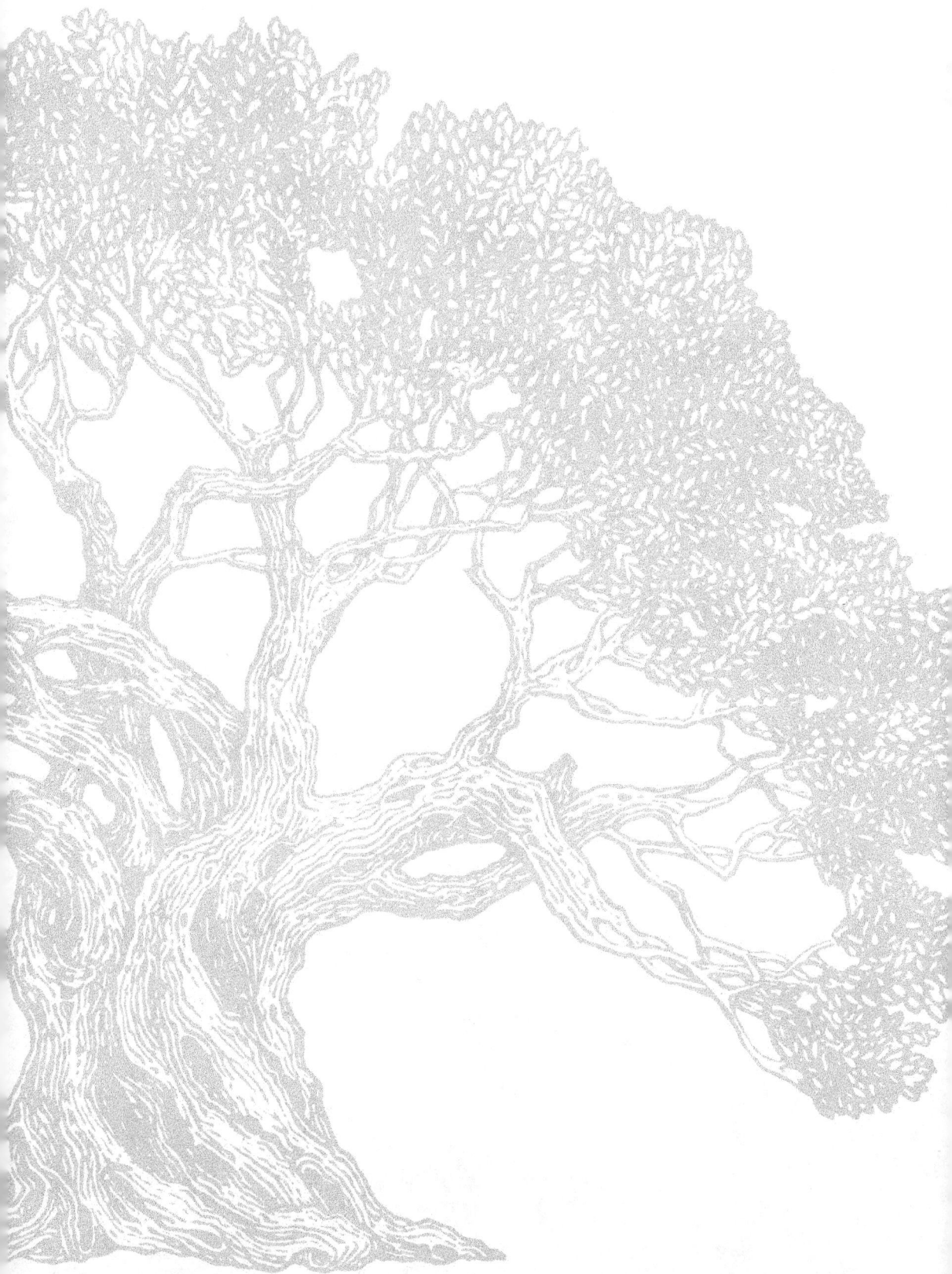

9

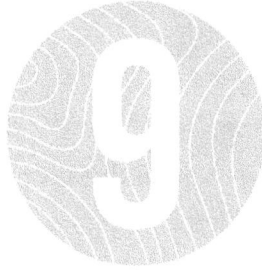

PRIMAL LIVING:
DESIGNING A LIFE WORTH LIVING

From Primal Reset to a Way of Life

The Primal Reset Program is not a quick-fix detox or a trendy wellness retreat where you sip green juice for a week and then return to the grind, none the wiser. No, this is your system reboot. It's a recalibration of your foundation for moving, eating, thinking, and living. Now, it's time to go deeper because the goal is not just to reset. The goal is to *live*.

Living primally isn't about chasing the latest health fads or clinging to outdated traditions. It's about mastering the art of adaptation, melding ancestral wisdom with the undeniable realities of the modern world. My time with the Hadzabe in the vast, sunbaked plains of East Africa taught me this firsthand. They don't merely survive in the wild; they thrive, seamlessly tuned to the rhythms of nature. Their movements, food, rest, and laughter all flow in sync, unburdened by the artificial constraints we've constructed for ourselves.

The irony? With all our technology, advancements, and conveniences, many of us have lost our primal intelligence. We live longer but *weaker*. More years, less vitality. And that, my friend, is not a trade worth making. This is where Primal Living comes in.

Remember Le Mans, the legendary 24-hour endurance race we opened the book with? Your life is not a drag race, a five-second burst of speed that burns out before the first curve. No, it is an endurance event, a test of resilience, efficiency, and precision. The objective isn't just to finish; it's to handle every turn, every challenge, every moment with mastery.

My background in neuroradiology has given me a front-row seat to witness what happens when we fail to respect this balance. Brains are prematurely aged by inflammation, and bodies are worn down by decades of quiet neglect. The scans don't lie, but they do point to the solution. We need to return to the core principles that made us strong in the first place.

My ancestors were woodworkers, shaping raw, untamed materials into something both functional and beautiful. That's what Primal Living is, crafting a life that isn't just long but rich in depth and meaning. It is about quantity *and* quality.

Your Primal Reset has opened the door. Now, it's time to walk through that door and never look back.

Maintaining a Lifetime of Peak Performance

In our 20s and 30s, we don't think about the long game. Performance is effortless. Reserves are overflowing. Our cognitive system hums like a finely tuned engine, our muscles respond without hesitation, and our joints feel indestructible. Because we *feel* good, we assume we *are* good. And that's where most people go wrong.

In those years, we don't see the slow undercurrent of decline. Sarcopenia begins in our 30s as muscles quietly slip away like sand through fingers. Joint mobility decreases if we don't deliberately maintain it. And the cognitive powerhouse we take for granted? After adulthood, we lose approximately 85,000 neurons per day. Let that sink in.

Unless we actively build new neuronal connections using the brain's capacity for neuroplasticity, we'll reach a point where focus dulls, memory recall slows, and mental sharpness fades. That's when people start complaining about brain fog, misplaced keys, and forgotten names. But that's not aging. It's *neglect*.

Emotional health follows the same trajectory. In our youth, life is structured—school, college, careers. There's always a syllabus, a checklist, and a boss dictating the next move. But if we don't define our purpose, we wake up one day, in a job, a life, a routine, without a *why*. That's when quiet desperation creeps in. That's when people start wondering, *Is this all there is?*

And then there's existential health, the final, often ignored pillar of a life well-lived. In the first half of life, we think we're invincible, the center of the universe. Mortality is a distant concept. Then, somewhere past middle age, reality catches up. If we haven't built a legacy mindset and invested in something greater than ourselves, the fear of mortality hits like a truck. But those who have devoted themselves to meaningful work, art, impact, and a cause that will outlive them? They find peace.

Consider me your halftime coach. Maybe the first half of your life wasn't optimized for performance. Perhaps you didn't know you needed to train for the long haul. But now you do. And we can still make the second half the best yet. With the right strategies, we don't just *extend* life, we maintain *vibrancy* throughout our years. That's the goal of this book. That's the promise of Primal Living.

Performance & Age

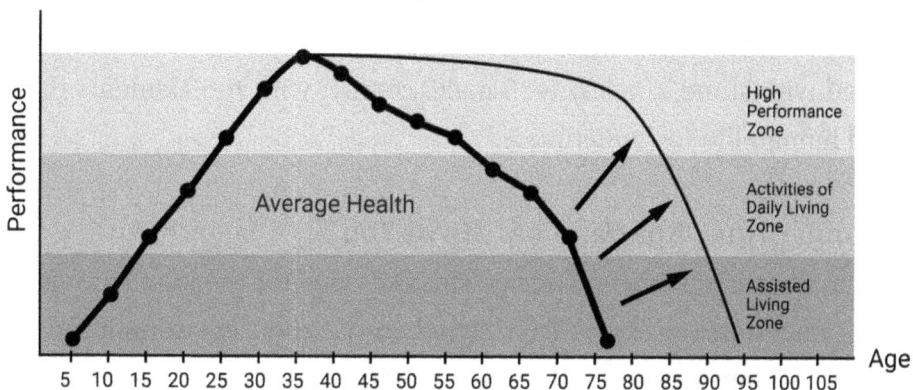

A Primal Home: A Blueprint for Longevity

Your home should be more than a shelter; it should be a living system that supports primal health. Every element, from the materials used to build and furnish a home to the design of the space, can either align with or disrupt our natural rhythms. A primal home is not a static structure but a living, breathing ecosystem that nurtures vitality, movement, and connection.

Earth Connection: Building with Nature

The Hadzabe understood the deep relationship between shelter and survival. Their homes were simple, temporary structures woven from branches and leaves, just enough to shield them from the elements while keeping them connected to the earth beneath their feet. There were no artificial barriers, no insulation from the rhythms of nature. Their bodies and minds adapted accordingly. Contrast that with the modern home: temperature-controlled, hermetically sealed, and often devoid of anything remotely organic.

To live primally, we must reclaim our connection to the earth. This involves incorporating natural materials such as stone, wood, clay, and even raw earth into our living spaces. It's about bringing the outside in: indoor plants that filter the air, wooden surfaces that retain warmth, and water features that add the soothing cadence of flowing nature.

But grounding isn't just about materials; it's about the physical act of connecting with the earth. A primal home should have spaces that invite you to be barefoot, allowing you to feel the texture of the ground and experience a moment of stillness as your body syncs with the planet's natural electromagnetic field. Whether it's a backyard with a small patch of wild grass or a meditation space lined with stone, the key is to make contact with the elements that have sustained human life for millennia.

Body Connection: Spaces That Move You

A body that does not move will decay. This is as true for the joints as it is for the mind. Our ancestors never needed a gym because their environment was their fitness center. They squatted, climbed, stretched, and ran for survival. But in today's world, we design homes for comfort, not for movement.

A primal home flips that script. Imagine spaces that encourage activity rather than passive existence: standing desks instead of chairs that invite hours of slumping, low tables, floor seating that keeps the hips and spine mobile, climbing holds along a hallway, a pull-up bar in a doorway, and an outdoor area designed for barefoot movement.

My grandfather, a master woodworker, built his home with an understanding of this principle—no rigid structures inhibited movement. His workspace was alive with tools, shelves placed at varying heights that required stretching and balance, an environment that demanded engagement rather than passive occupation. Your home can do the same.

Food Connection: Designing for Nutritional Intelligence

The modern kitchen is a paradox. It is filled with appliances that speed up food preparation, yet most people spend less time cooking than ever before. A primal kitchen is not just a place to prepare meals, it is a space that fosters a relationship with real food.

Imagine a fermentation station where kefir and kombucha brew in glass jars, reminding you that gut health requires ongoing attention. A countertop garden with fresh herbs ready to be plucked. An open shelving system that prioritizes whole ingredients, including grains, nuts, and dried fruits, over the processed foods that lurk behind cupboard doors.

Your kitchen should be an invitation to nourish yourself. Instead of a microwave-centered layout, a primal kitchen has a central cooking area that encourages ritual. A wood-burning stove or even an outdoor cooking space brings back the sensory engagement of preparing meals with fire and earth.

Mind Connection: Creating Spaces for Mental Clarity

We all know firsthand the effects of overstimulation on the brain. The constant flood of artificial light, digital screens, and clutter disrupts cognitive function. A primal home must counteract this.

Quiet zones are essential; they are dedicated spaces free of screens, where the nervous system can relax and downshift from a state of high alert. Lighting should mimic the sun's natural rhythms: dim and warm in the evening, bright and blue-tinted in the morning. Walls painted in earthy, muted tones offer a visual sense of calm.

Even sound design matters. Water features, wind chimes, or simply the absence of electronic noise can shape how we think and feel. Just as the Hadzabe sat around the fire in reflective silence after a long day of hunting, we must create environments that allow the mind to settle, process, and renew.

Purpose & Community: A Home for Connection

A primal home is not just about the individual but about the collective. In Asian Indian culture, the home is a multi-generational space where storytelling, wisdom, and shared experience shape identity.

Open spaces designed for gathering—a communal table, a fire pit, a storytelling corner—bring back the tradition of human connection. My grandmother's home was never quiet; it was filled with voices, debates, laughter, and the rhythmic chopping of vegetables in the kitchen. In contrast, many modern homes are designed for isolation, featuring separate rooms, personal screens, and closed doors. We must reverse this trend.

Mortality & Cosmos: Designing for Legacy

We are mortal, but how we live with that truth determines the quality of our days. Most modern homes are designed to avoid this reality; there is no space for contemplation, no acknowledgment of impermanence.

A primal home embraces mortality as an integral part of its design. It has art that depicts cycles of nature. It has spaces for reflection: meditation corners, altars, or even a simple window strategically placed to frame the stars at night, reminding us of our place in the vastness of existence. In the second half of life, our focus shifts from accumulation to legacy. A home should reflect that transition, offering a space to live and create a legacy.

Your home is not just where you live, it is where you thrive. Every choice in its design should serve your highest vitality. From the materials that touch your skin to the movement patterns it encourages, from the food it nurtures to the connections it fosters, a primal home is a blueprint for longevity.

We cannot control time, but we can control how we live within it. A home designed with primal intelligence does more than shelter us; it aligns us with the most resounding rhythms of life, ensuring that we move, think, eat, and connect in ways that allow us to flourish.

Mastering the Digital Age Without Letting It Master Us

The Hadzabe taught me something profound: No tribal member stares at glowing rectangles. Their lives are not dominated by beeping notifications, endless scrolling, or the dopamine rush of social media likes. Instead, their attention is fully absorbed in the real world: tracking animals, deciphering the whispers of the wind, listening to the stories of their elders by firelight. Compare that to the modern scene of a family at dinner, each person glued to their screen, bodies present but minds elsewhere.

Technology is a tool, but it must serve us, not the other way around. **Our primal ancestors were toolmakers, not slaves to tools.** My grandfather understood this intuitively. The chisel didn't dictate his work; he controlled it and wielded it with intention. It's time we did the same with our devices.

Tech Fasting: Reclaiming Attention

Fasting isn't just for food. We need digital fasts, intentional screen-free zones, and hours when our brains recalibrate to a pre-Internet baseline. Think about it: When was the last time you sat in silence, truly present, letting your thoughts stretch and breathe?

The brain, much like the body, needs cycles of engagement and recovery. We have seen the effects of chronic digital stimulation: fragmented attention, decreased cognitive resilience, and structural brain changes linked to addiction-like behaviors. The constant influx of information hijacks the brain's default mode network, which is responsible for deep thinking and self-reflection. **If you're constantly consuming, when do you create?**

Consider tech fasting in layers:

- **Micro-fasts:** No screens for the first and last hour of your day.

- **Tech-free zones:** Designate a room in your home as a screen-free sanctuary: no phones, no TVs, just real human connection.

- **Deep fasts:** One entire weekend a month, fully unplug. No texts, no emails, no screens. Just you and the analog world.

Primal Workflows: Designing for Deep Focus

Technology should enhance productivity, not fragment it. However, modern workspaces are digital battlegrounds, constantly bombarded by emails, pings, and algorithmically optimized distractions. The result? A cognitive drain that leaves us exhausted yet unfulfilled, busy yet ineffective.

The solution? Primal workflows.

1. **Batching and Deep Work:** Instead of constant task-switching (which burns through mental energy like a leaky faucet), set aside dedicated blocks for deep, uninterrupted work. No notifications, no email checking. Protect this time fiercely.

2. **Single-Tasking Mastery:** Our ancestors weren't scanning six tabs at once while hunting an antelope. They were fully engaged in the task at hand. The brain thrives on focus. Train it by committing to single-tasking, whether reading, writing, or problem-solving.

3. **Movement-Based Thinking:** My best ideas don't come while I'm staring at a screen; they emerge during a long walk, in the middle of a workout, or while working with my hands. Physical

movement fuels cognitive breakthroughs. Incorporate walking meetings, standing desks, or sprints during work.

AI and the Mind: Outsourcing Efficiency, Not Intelligence

AI is here to stay. It can accelerate efficiency, automate menial tasks, and even augment creativity. But it must never replace our primal intelligence, our ability to think critically, connect deeply, and problem-solve in intuitive ways no machine can.

Outsource wisely. Utilize AI for what it excels at: organization, automation, and streamlining repetitive tasks. But don't let it think for you.

A calculator won't make you better at mental math. Similarly, relying on AI for every decision atrophies our cognitive abilities. Instead, use it as an ally, not a crutch.

- **Enhance, don't replace:** Let AI handle scheduling, data sorting, and email filtering, but keep your brain sharp by engaging in fundamental analysis, creativity, and strategy.

- **Protect your mind's playground:** AI can generate but not imagine. The most valuable mental work (innovation, intuition, insight) comes from a well-trained, actively engaged brain.

- **Set clear boundaries:** Limit AI-driven decision-making in areas that require deep human understanding, such as relationships, leadership, and creative work.

The Future is Analog AND Digital

The key to mastering technology is balance. We are not meant to live in a purely digital world, just as we are not meant to reject AI entirely. The Hadza do not need smartphones, but they also don't perform complex neurosurgery. We exist at the intersection of primal wisdom and modern innovation. The challenge is to wield both skillfully.

So, the choice is yours. Let the glowing rectangles own your mind or take back control and use them as the powerful tools they are meant to be. Like my grandfather's chisel, they are only as valuable as the hands guiding them.

Primal Neighborhoods: Reclaiming the Village Mindset

The nuclear family is a modern failed experiment, an artificial construct that isolates us from the support systems that sustained our ancestors for thousands of years. Humans were never meant to live in single-family silos, peering at the world through the narrow frame of a backyard fence. We are wired for community, the organic give-and-take of shared spaces, and the kind of human connection that doesn't require an RSVP. The Hadzabe didn't need to schedule playdates or block parties; every meal, every story, every fire was a communal event. That was life, and it worked.

Modern society, however, has drifted far from this primal blueprint. Today, we design neighborhoods that prioritize cars over people, security over spontaneity, and convenience over connection. If we want to reclaim our ancestors' vitality, resilience, and longevity, we must rethink how we build our communities. The key is not just in how we design our homes but in how we structure the spaces between them. A primal neighborhood fosters movement, interaction, and self-sufficiency; it is one where older adults are not warehoused, children are not sequestered, and nature is not an afterthought.

Walkability and Nature Access: Making Movement Natural

A primal neighborhood is one where walking is not a chore but a way of life. In the villages of India where my ancestors once lived, no one needed a gym membership. Physical activity was built into the rhythm of daily existence. Compare that to the modern suburban landscape, where a trip to the grocery store means getting into a car, sidewalks are decorative rather than functional, and green spaces are something we "visit" rather than inhabit.

Walkability isn't just about exercise; it's about engagement. When people walk, they see each other. They exchange nods, stop for conversation, and take note of the subtle changes in their surroundings. Trails, parks, and communal green spaces should be as essential as roads, integral arteries of human connection. And let's not forget nature. We need trees that provide shade, gardens that supply food, and water features that invite reflection. The closer we can live in harmony with the natural world, the more aligned we are with the rhythms that sustain our health.

Shared Spaces: Bringing Back the Village Fire

The Hadza sit around a fire every night, telling stories, laughing, and reinforcing the bonds that make survival possible. In contrast, modern neighborhoods are built for separation. We retreat behind walls, binge-watch alone, and rely on scheduled social interactions. This isn't just unnatural, it's unhealthy.

To build a primal neighborhood, we must design for gathering. Fire pits, communal gardens, and outdoor kitchens invite people to linger, share, and break bread together. The Mediterranean concept of the "piazza" or the Indian village "chowk" are not just town squares; they are the heartbeats of their communities. We need modern equivalents, places where neighbors can interact spontaneously, without the artificiality of planned events. Because community isn't built in scheduled increments, it grows in the everyday moments of unplanned connection.

Intergenerational Living: The Wisdom of the Old, the Energy of the Young

Societies with the longest lifespans and best health share a crucial trait: they promote **intergenerational integration.** The young and the old do not live in separate orbits. In traditional cultures, older adults are not sidelined; they are honored, sought after for their guidance, and remain active participants in the community's daily affairs. When aging is treated as a medical condition rather than a life stage, cognitive decline accelerates, loneliness deepens, and purpose fades.

Imagine a neighborhood where children play freely under the watchful eyes of wise elders, where storytelling bridges the past and the future, where aging is not something to be feared but is instead embraced as a life stage of deep significance. We need multi-generational housing models that foster interaction rather than isolation. Instead of senior living communities that function as waiting rooms for decline, we need living spaces that foster purpose, mentorship, and intergenerational connection.

Self-Sufficiency & Resilience: Beyond Consumer Culture

A primal neighborhood is not dependent on endless supply chains and outside resources, it is built on local resilience. My grandfather, a skilled woodworker, didn't buy furniture from a store; he crafted it with his own hands, selecting the wood, shaping it, and creating something that would last a lifetime. We have lost this self-reliance in our hyper-consumptive culture, but it is something we can regain.

Neighborhoods should have access to shared resources, including community gardens that provide fresh food, tool libraries that reduce waste, and regenerative farming initiatives that help rebuild the soil. Instead of being passive consumers, we should be active participants in creating what sustains us. This shift isn't just about survival, it's about empowerment. When people have a hand in producing their food, building their own spaces, and contributing to their community's well-being, they gain a deeper sense of purpose and fulfillment.

Reclaiming the Village Mindset

At its core, a primal neighborhood is not just about better urban planning, it's about reclaiming the essence of what it means to be human. It's about moving away from isolation and toward interdependence. It's about designing spaces that foster longevity, not just in years but in quality of life. We must recognize that health isn't just about what we eat or how we exercise. It's about where and how we live. The village mindset isn't an outdated relic; it's the missing link to a life that is long, rich, meaningful, and deeply connected.

The way forward isn't just about reclaiming our health, it's about reclaiming our humanity. And that starts with where we live, who we surround ourselves with, and how we build the spaces that shape our lives.

Primal Kids: Teaching the Next Generation How to Live

Children today are growing up in a world designed for convenience, comfort, and, ironically, disconnection. The Hadzabe children didn't need playgrounds; the world was their playground. They climbed trees to chase birds, ran barefoot over rough terrain without flinching, and learned to wield a bow before they could even spell their names. Compare that to modern children, strapped into car seats, glued to screens, and hovering under an umbrella of constant parental supervision.

We are raising a generation that knows more about YouTube influencers than their ancestral roots. They are drowning in artificial environments, processed foods, and dopamine-driven distractions. If we are serious about longevity, we cannot ignore the future, our children. We must return them to real life. We must teach them to move, build, embrace risk, and connect in ways that no touchscreen ever can.

Let Them Move

The human body is a primal machine built for movement, not passive existence. Watch a toddler before society tells them how to behave; they squat perfectly, climb instinctively, and run before they can talk in complete sentences. Then we shove them into chairs for eight hours a day and wonder why they lose their flexibility and strength.

Barefoot time isn't a hippie fantasy; it's biomechanics. Walking barefoot strengthens the foot's arches, improves balance, and enhances proprioception, our body's natural GPS. Yet today's kids grow up in stiff, over-padded shoes that disconnect them from the earth beneath them. Let them run barefoot on grass, feel the cold of river water on their toes, and climb trees where their ancestors once sought refuge.

Schools teach children that movement is something to be contained: sit still, don't fidget, stay in line. However, primal children need more than 30 minutes of recess and ways to engage their whole bodies. Let them crawl, climb, and leap from rocks. Give them spaces to swing, hang, and balance. The Hadza never had a "leg day."They had a life of movement. And that's how it should be.

Let Them Build

My grandfather's workshop smelled of sawdust and sweat; it was a sacred space where raw wood was transformed into something both functional and beautiful. That was my classroom before school ever was. My hands learned the language of tools, the feel of grain direction, and the patience that comes with craftsmanship.

Today's kids? They swipe, tap, and consume. Their thumbs are strong from gaming, but their hands are weak from a lack of real-world experience. If you want a child to understand creativity, don't give them another app; provide them with a hammer.

Let them build. Woodworking, stone sculpting, and metal forging are skills that connect us to our lineage as makers, not just consumers. In India, my ancestors carved intricate designs into temple doors, each chisel mark a meditation. In neuroscience, we understand that hands-on engagement strengthens the mind by forming new neural pathways in ways that passive screen consumption cannot.

When children learn to build something with their hands, they gain more than just a skill; they develop self-reliance, problem-solving abilities, and patience. Give a child a plank of wood and a set of nails, and they might build a bench. But more importantly, they will certainly build confidence.

Let Them Experience Risk

The modern world has sterilized childhood, padding it with safety rails and participation trophies. But resilience is not born in comfort; it is forged in challenge.

The Hadza children I knew didn't just play, they engaged in controlled risk-taking. They learned to navigate thorny bushes, handle fire, and test their limits without an adult stepping in every two minutes. They understood that failure was an integral part of learning, not something to be avoided; it was a necessary step in the process.

Yet in today's world, we sanitize childhood experiences to the point where a scraped knee is a crisis. Parents hover like overprotective drones, ensuring their kids never stumble, physically or emotionally. However, a child who never faces a struggle will never develop strength.

Let them fall. Let them climb too high, miscalculate a jump, or attempt something that scares them. Risk teaches consequence. It sharpens instincts. A child who learns to embrace controlled adversity today will grow into an adult who can navigate real-world challenges tomorrow.

Let Them Connect

A child without connection is a ship without a compass. Connection is not found in Wi-Fi signals but in the wisdom of elders, the bonds of community, and the rituals that remind us we are part of something greater than ourselves.

In India, storytelling is a tradition inherited through generations, wisdom wrapped in parables and poetry. Parents alone didn't raise the neighborhood children I knew; they were raised by the village, by the elders who carried the memory of the land. They sat around fires listening to stories of ancestors, learning who they were by understanding where they came from.

Compare that to the modern family, where dinner is eaten in separate rooms, and the only fires we sit around are the ones flickering on our screens. Children need elders, rituals, and a sense of belonging. If we do not provide them with that, they will seek connection in shallow places, such as social media validation, fleeting digital trends, and artificial communities that lack genuine substance.

Bring back the family meal. Create spaces for deep conversations. Let children listen to their grandparents' stories and learn the wisdom carried in their wrinkles. Teach them that life is not just about individual success but about contributing to something bigger than themselves.

If we want the next generation to thrive, we must stop raising them like domesticated pets and start raising them like primal humans. A child who moves freely, builds fearlessly, embraces challenge, and connects deeply is a child who will carry the torch of longevity into the future.

We inherit the earth from our ancestors and must protect it for our children. If we want them to reclaim their primal health, we must first show them how to live it. The path to longevity does not begin in adulthood, it starts in childhood. And it begins with us.

Breathspan: The True Measure of Longevity

In the ancient wisdom of India, lifespan is not measured in years, but in breaths. The concept of *prana*, or life force, suggests that each of us is allotted a finite number of breaths from birth. The slower and deeper we breathe, the longer we live. This idea, which may seem mystical at first, aligns remarkably well with modern scientific principles. Our breath is more than just an automatic function; it is the gateway to our nervous system, our healthspan, and ultimately, our longevity.

The average human at rest breathes about 12 to 20 breaths per minute. That equates to roughly 17,000 to 30,000 breaths per day. However, individuals with lower baseline respiratory rates, such as elite endurance athletes, meditation practitioners, and centenarians, often breathe at 6 to 10 breaths per minute, effectively halving their total breath count over a lifetime.

Physiologically, a lower respiratory rate is directly correlated with increased parasympathetic tone, which activates our body's "rest and digest" state. This shift reduces inflammation, decreases oxidative stress, and enhances cardiovascular efficiency. In contrast, chronic shallow breathing, a hallmark of modern stress, keeps us locked in a sympathetic, fight-or-flight state, accelerating cellular aging.

Modern research on respiration supports what Indian traditions have known for millennia: Slowing the breath slows down the aging process. Studies have shown that lower resting respiratory rates are associated with improved heart rate variability (HRV), reduced cortisol levels, and increased resistance to disease. The longest-living creatures on Earth, the giant tortoises, whales, and elephants, have the lowest resting respiratory rates. The Greenland shark, which can live for over 400 years, breathes at an imperceptibly slow rate. In contrast, animals with rapid, shallow breaths, like mice, live only a few years.

Humans fall somewhere in between, but the lesson remains:

The more efficiently we breathe, the longer and healthier we live.

Every primal practice we've explored in this book, including connecting with **earth, body, food, mind, purpose, community, and finiteness,** leads to one central outcome: a calmer, more efficient system. When we align with these natural rhythms, our **inflammation drops, our nervous system rebalances, and our breath slows.** This is the essence of expanding our breathspan.

- **Earth Connection** – Grounding in nature naturally deepens our breath, stabilizing the nervous system.

- **Body Connection** – Movement, especially slow and controlled exercise like yoga or resistance training, teaches breath control and efficiency.

- **Food Connection** – Consuming whole, anti-inflammatory foods reduces metabolic stress, allowing for deeper, unlabored breaths.

- **Mind Connection** – Meditation and mindfulness practices have been shown to lower respiratory rates by increasing vagal tone, thereby promoting a sense of calm and well-being.

- **Purpose & Community** – A life filled with meaning and social connection reduces anxiety, which in turn slows respiration.

- **Finiteness** – Accepting mortality and cultivating inner stillness helps lower stress, guiding us toward effortless, long, and deep breaths.

At the core of *Primal Health Design* is a simple truth: The more efficient your system becomes, the lower your resting respiratory rate and the greater your breathspan. Breathspan is the hidden metric behind longevity. It is the ultimate indicator of how well you are truly living.

As a radiologist, I have spent decades observing how these fundamental practices affect the human brain and body. As a child, I witnessed the Hadza living with effortless grace, their breath in sync with the rhythms of nature. As the descendant of woodworkers, I understand that perfection is found in simplicity; just as a finely-crafted piece of wood has no wasted material, a well-lived life has no wasted breath.

This book is not just a guide; it is an invitation to reclaim your breath. To slow down, not in the sense of doing less, but in the sense of living more deeply. Because in the end, longevity is not simply about extending time, it is about filling each breath with meaning, health, and presence.

So, take a deep breath.

And begin.

Living Primal and Fulfilled

To live primally is to live awake. Feel the earth beneath your feet, the fire in your belly, and the rhythm of your breath in sync with the rising and setting sun. It is to move with purpose, eat with intention, think with clarity, and love with depth. **It is to break free from the numbing comforts of modernity and reclaim what was always ours—the birthright of a life fully lived.**

The Hadzabe live without alarms, notifications, or schedules, yet they manage their time efficiently. They hunt, gather, laugh, and tell stories with a presence that most of us lost the moment we first stared into a glowing screen. My ancestors carved masterpieces not by chasing perfection but by honoring the rawness of the grain, the unpredictability of the knots, the story that each piece of wood carried. It is in this rawness, this embrace of imperfection, that true fulfillment is found.

My life has been the intersection of tradition and innovation. Raised in an Asian Indian household, I was immersed in a culture that valued both intellect and intuition. My childhood in Africa taught me the power of simplicity, how health and happiness stem not from excess but from alignment with nature. Later, as a neuroradiologist, I had the opportunity to peer into the human body, reading the whispers of aging brains and degenerating bones. Each path I've walked has led me to this conclusion:

Health is not just about avoiding disease but about crafting a life of resilience, passion, and purpose.

The patterns are undeniable—atrophy where movement was abandoned, decay where nourishment was neglected, and decline where curiosity was stifled. But the good news? None of it is inevitable. A primal life is a choice. A choice to move daily, to eat food that still remembers the soil, to stretch the mind with new ideas, to forge deep connections, and to stare into the cosmos with a sense of reverence rather than insignificance.

This book serves as a blueprint for those who seek to design their own primal life. It is not about rigid rules or ascetic living but about integrating health-supporting elements into the spaces where we live, work, and play. Your home should nourish your body, your workspace should enhance your focus, and your daily routines should foster vitality. Primal living is about making intentional choices, choosing real food over processed convenience foods, opting for movement over stagnation, prioritizing relationships over digital distractions, and embracing purpose over a passive existence.

Living primally is not about rejecting modernity but about mastering it. It's about using technology without becoming its servant, building wealth without sacrificing time, and extending life not just in years, but in vibrancy as well. It is about knowing, at the end of each day, that we did not just exist but truly lived.

A fulfilled life is not measured in years but in depth. The goal is not merely longevity but presence, impact, and legacy. When you live primally, you live deeply. You breathe the wild air, sweat under the sun, stand tall in adversity, and love with an intensity that leaves echoes long after you are gone.

So, go. Live primally. Live deeply. Live fully.

ACKNOWLEDGEMENTS

My Parents

I dedicate this book to my parents, Dalpat and Sudha Mistry, the original architects of my life, and the quiet, enduring inspiration behind *Primal Health Design*.

My deepest regret is that I wasn't able to place this book in their hands while they were still here. My mom passed away a year and a half before my dad, and he followed her a little over a year prior to this book's publication. And yet even in their passing, they left me with lessons I could never have learned in a classroom. The paradigm I explore in this book about connecting with our finiteness, how mortality clarifies what matters most, was etched into my soul through the grief of losing them both.

My father's work as a civil engineer with the UN World Bank took us across continents, to Tanzania and beyond. His sense of wonder opened doors most children never get to walk through. Because of him, I stood among the Hadzabe tribe in Africa, played under baobab trees, and learned early that life is bigger, deeper, and more connected than textbooks tell you.

But my parents' greatest gift wasn't a destination, it was how they let me experience the world. We moved more than 22 times during my childhood. At the time, it felt like a burden: another move, another goodbye. But looking back, I see it now as the greatest education I could have asked for. Each home, each culture, each environment planted seeds in me that would one day bloom into this work.

Growing up, I took so many things for granted. The Indian cultural rituals my mom practiced daily were just background noise at the time. But now, I recognize them as the sacred rhythm of wisdom, of nourishment, of knowing how to live in sync with the earth. She was the keeper of traditions I now carry forward.

And my dad. He may have worked in concrete and blueprints, but his heart never left the family lineage of woodworking. He built small furniture pieces around the house, always with intention and care. In every design he created, there was a principle at play: function, form, and feeling. Today, I design health systems with the same spirit: practical, beautiful, and built to last.

Mom. Dad. Everything I am is because of you. This book, this mission, this message—it's yours. Thank you for raising me not just to think, but to feel. Not just to know, but to live.

Hetal

We met in our twenties, but in truth, we've grown up together. In those early years, we didn't yet know what life would ask of us, only that we'd face it side by side. Through every season, medical school's relentless pace, residency's exhausting nights, and the demanding world of neuroradiology, you stood by me with strength, laughter, and a kind of knowing that never wavered.

I've spent years immersed in anatomy, health, and the science of longevity. But you've always had the deeper wisdom, knowing the art of living well. You've reminded me, time and time again, that healing is not just a process of the body, but a rhythm of the soul.

Since the age of three, you knew you were an artist. That's not a line, it's a legacy. While most people spend their entire lives trying to find their purpose, you've been living yours, brushstroke by brushstroke, creating from a space of wonder. Your creations don't just decorate space, they heal it. They speak in the language of color, texture, and nature, and they say what words often cannot.

Everything I do, I do for you. And not in some grand, romantic gesture, but in the most practical and profound way. You've made the abstract real. You've given my work its soul. You are the reason I understand the deeper "why" behind health, behind beauty, behind balance.

Primal Health Design is a book about reconnection to nature, to purpose, to breath, to stillness, to vitality. And you, Hetal, embody every one of these elements. You are grounded and ethereal, timeless and fully present, wild and wise. You are the gentle reminder that amidst all the technology, complexity, and speed of this world, there is still a place for slowness, softness, and soul.

Thank you for walking with me through all versions of myself. Thank you for believing in this vision even before it had a name. You are the center of my compass, the rhythm in my breath, and the design behind everything I create.

Om

Om, as a son, you've been one of life's greatest blessings, a living thread in the lineage of creators, craftsmen, and thinkers that runs through our family's history. You carry the spirit of our woodworker ancestry, not just in hands that can shape and build, but in a mind that designs with clarity, purpose, and beauty.

You are wise beyond your years. You seem to straddle two worlds with ease, honoring ancient values while navigating the complexities of modern technology like a seasoned strategist. You're the family's think tank, the quiet architect of brilliant ideas, and the first one I turn to when I need a fresh, fearless perspective.

Sometimes, I look at your discipline and marvel. It outpaces even mine (and trust me, that's not easy to admit). As a college student, you've stayed true to your heart and purpose, refusing to follow someone else's script. Everything you touch reflects a quiet excellence—never loud, always luminous.

In God's time, I have no doubt you'll rise as a powerful entrepreneur and creator. But more importantly, you'll do it with character, clarity, and kindness. We can't wait to see the world you'll build with that rare blend of intellect, intuition, and heart.

Sai

Sai, you are the spiritual anchor in my life, the stillness in the storm, the reminder of what truly matters. Every time I look into your eyes, I see something ancient, a depth of truth that's rare, especially in someone your age. You walk through high school halls with the presence of an old soul, quietly watching, deeply feeling, and intuitively knowing.

You see the world through a different lens, one that doesn't blur with noise or distraction. And while that may set you apart now, I know that in time, your light will draw others toward you. There's a primal intelligence within you that will unfold exactly as it's meant to, and when it does, people will be better for having known you.

You are the warrior in our family, not in the loud, brash sense but in the quiet courage you carry. You're bold where I was once hesitant. Fearless, while others are still finding their footing. Never lose that strength. It will guide you through life's mountains and valleys with clarity and conviction.

Sai, I know you'll be a great coach and mentor to others. Your insight, your fire, your stillness are a gift. And the world needs more of what you carry.

Ronak

Ronak, as a brother, you've always been the steady hand, anchoring our family with your quiet strength and unwavering presence. Thank you for being close to Mom and Dad, especially in their final years. Your support meant more than words can capture.

Now, as we carry their legacy forward, I see in you the same values they cherished: loyalty, humility, and heart. You're a good husband, a loving father, and a deeply creative soul. That creativity is your spark; don't ever lose it. And your calm, grounded presence? That's your superpower. We may walk different paths, but I'll always be grateful that you walk beside me.

Tanya

Tanya, as an editor, you took me in as a first-time author and, with quiet strength, helped me grow. You didn't just edit my words, you shaped my confidence. There were moments I doubted my voice, thinking, *Who's going to read this stuff?* But you gently reminded me, *"No—the world needs this."*

That single sentence carried me through so many chapters.

Your insight, your calm encouragement, your ability to see the essence beneath the rough draft; I've trusted your perspective every step of the way. This book wouldn't exist in its current form without you. I couldn't have done it without your steady hand and open heart.

REFERENCES

Introduction:

Lifespan versus healthspan: Seals, D. R., Justice, J. N., & LaRocca, T. J. (2016). Physiological geroscience: targeting function to increase healthspan and achieve optimal longevity. The Journal of physiology, 594(8), 2001–2024. https://doi.org/10.1113/jphysiol.2014.282665

Average life expectancy: Centers for Disease Control and Prevention. (n.d.). Life expectancy. National Center for Health Statistics. https://www.cdc.gov/nchs/fastats/life-expectancy.htm

Obesity rate: Centers for Disease Control and Prevention. (2024). Prevalence of obesity among adults and youth: United States, 2021–2022 (NCHS Data Brief No. 508). National Center for Health Statistics.https://www.cdc.gov/nchs/data/databriefs/db508.pdf

Suicide rate: Centers for Disease Control and Prevention. (n.d.). Suicide data and statistics. National Center for Injury Prevention and Control. https://www.cdc.gov/suicide/facts/data.html

Rising rate of mental health issues: National Institute of Mental Health. (n.d.). Mental illness: Statistics. U.S. Department of Health and Human Services. https://www.nimh.nih.gov/health/statistics/mental-illness

Homo sapiens, as a species, have roamed this earth for approximately 300,000 years: Mcbrearty, S., & Brooks, A. S. (2000). The revolution that wasn't: a new interpretation of the origin of modern human behavior. Journal of human evolution, 39(5), 453–563. https://doi.org/10.1006/jhev.2000.0435

The Hadzabe people have inhabited the region surrounding Lake Eyasi: Marlowe, F. W. (2010). The Hadza: Hunter-Gatherers of Tanzania. Univ. of California Press.

Emerging comprehensive biological aging model: Hamczyk, M. R., Nevado, R. M., Barettino, A., Fuster, V., & Andrés, V. (2020). Biological Versus Chronological Aging: JACC Focus Seminar. Journal of the American College of Cardiology, 75(8), 919–930. https://doi.org/10.1016/j.jacc.2019.11.062

24 Hours of Le Mans: Le Mans: Spurring, Q. (2011). Le Mans 1930-39: The official history of the world's greatest motor race. Evro Publishing.

Chapter 1

Direct contact with the earth allows the transfer of electrons from the ground into the body:

Chevalier, G., Sinatra, S. T., Oschman, J. L., Sokal, K., & Sokal, P. (2012). Earthing: health implications of reconnecting the human body to the Earth's surface electrons. Journal of environmental and public health, 2012, 291541. https://doi.org/10.1155/2012/291541

Grounding: Sinatra, S. T., Sinatra, D. S., Sinatra, S. W., & Chevalier, G. (2023). Grounding - The universal anti-inflammatory remedy. Biomedical journal, 46(1), 11–16. https://doi.org/10.1016/j.bj.2022.12.002

Subjects who slept on grounded conductive mats were found to have reduced levels of inflammation-related biomarkers: Oschman, J. L., Chevalier, G., & Brown, R. (2015). The effects of grounding (earthing) on inflammation, the immune response, wound healing, and prevention and treatment of chronic inflammatory and autoimmune diseases. Journal of inflammation research, 8, 83–96. https://doi.org/10.2147/JIR.S69656

Walking barefoot increases proprioceptive input, enhances motor control, and reduces fall risk: Lieberman D. E. (2012). What we can learn about running from barefoot running: an evolutionary medical perspective. Exercise and sport sciences reviews, 40(2), 63–72. https://doi.org/10.1097/JES.0b013e31824ab210

Barefoot walking and minimalist footwear significantly activate intrinsic foot muscles: Ridge, S. T., Olsen, M. T., Bruening, D. A., Jurgensmeier, K., Griffin, D., Davis, I. S., & Johnson, A. W. (2019). Walking in Minimalist Shoes Is Effective for Strengthening Foot Muscles. Medicine and science in sports and exercise, 51(1), 104–113. https://doi.org/10.1249/MSS.0000000000001751

Barefoot walking improves reaction time and spatial awareness: Menant, J. C., Steele, J. R., Menz, H. B., Munro, B. J., & Lord, S. R. (2008). Optimizing footwear for older people at risk of falls. Journal of rehabilitation research and development, 45(8), 1167–1181.

A time capsule for foot evolution: McNutt, E. J., Zipfel, B., & DeSilva, J. M. (2018). The evolution of the human foot. Evolutionary anthropology, 27(5), 197–217. https://doi.org/10.1002/evan.21713

Flat arch: Saldías, E., Malgosa, A., Jordana, X., Martínez-Labarga, C., Coppa, A., Rubini, M., Vila, B., & Isidro, A. (2021). A new methodology to estimate flat foot in skeletal remains - the example of Mediterranean collections. Homo : internationale Zeitschrift fur die vergleichende Forschung am Menschen, 72(4), 281–292. https://doi.org/10.1127/homo/2021/1320

Modern footwear has increased the incidence of conditions such as plantar fasciitis: Sichting, F., Holowka, N. B., Hansen, O. B., & Lieberman, D. E. (2020). Effect of the upward curvature of toe springs on walking biomechanics in humans. Scientific reports, 10(1), 14643. https://doi.org/10.1038/s41598-020-71247-9

Shinrin-Yoku: Park, B. J., Tsunetsugu, Y., Kasetani, T., Kagawa, T., & Miyazaki, Y. (2010). The physiological effects of Shinrin-yoku (taking in the forest atmosphere or forest bathing): evidence from field experiments in 24 forests across Japan. Environmental health and preventive medicine, 15(1), 18–26. https://doi.org/10.1007/s12199-009-0086-9

Forest Bathing: Qing Li. Forest Bathing: How Trees Can Help You Find Health and Happiness. Viking, 2018.

Health-promoting phytoncides: Li Q. (2010). Effect of forest bathing trips on human immune function. Environmental health and preventive medicine, 15(1), 9–17. https://doi.org/10.1007/s12199-008-0068-3

Environments rich in negative ions can influence our health: Xiao, S., Wei, T., Petersen, J. D., Zhou, J., & Lu, X. (2023). Biological effects of negative air ions on human health and integrated multiomics to identify biomarkers: a literature review. Environmental science and pollution research international, 30(27), 69824–69836. https://doi.org/10.1007/s11356-023-27133-8

Air ions, mood and overall well-being: Goel, N., & Etwaroo, G. R. (2006). Bright light, negative air ions, and auditory stimuli produce rapid mood changes in a student population: a placebo-controlled study. Psychological medicine, 36(9), 1253–1263. https://doi.org/10.1017/S0033291706008002

Negative ions improve respiratory function: Liu, S., Huang, Q., Wu, Y., Song, Y., Dong, W., Chu, M., Yang, D., Zhang, X., Zhang, J., Chen, C., Zhao, B., Shen, H., Guo, X., & Deng, F. (2020). Metabolic linkages between indoor negative air ions, particulate matter and cardiorespiratory function: A randomized, double-blind crossover study among children. Environment international, 138, 105663. https://doi.org/10.1016/j.envint.2020.105663

Exposure to natural environments and mental health improvement: Bratman, G. N., Hamilton, J. P., & Daily, G. C. (2012). The impacts of nature experience on human cognitive function and mental health. Annals of the New York Academy of Sciences, 1249, 118–136. https://doi.org/10.1111/j.1749-6632.2011.06400.x

Immersing ourselves in nature invigorates our neural pathways: Bratman, G. N., Anderson, C. B., Berman, M. G., Cochran, B., de Vries, S., Flanders, J., Folke, C., Frumkin, H., Gross, J. J., Hartig, T., Kahn, P. H., Jr, Kuo, M., Lawler, J. J., Levin, P. S., Lindahl, T., Meyer-Lindenberg, A., Mitchell, R., Ouyang, Z., Roe, J., Scarlett, L., ... Daily, G. C. (2019). Nature and mental health: An ecosystem service perspective. Science advances, 5(7), eaax0903. https://doi.org/10.1126/sciadv.aax0903

Nature nurtures our cognitive resources: Berman, M. G., Jonides, J., & Kaplan, S. (2008). The cognitive benefits of interacting with nature. Psychological science, 19(12), 1207–1212. https://doi.org/10.1111/j.1467-9280.2008.02225.x

Nature and BDNF levels: Park SA, Son SY, Lee AY, Park HG, Lee WL, Lee CH. Park, S. A., Son, S. Y., Lee, A. Y., Park, H. G., Lee, W. L., & Lee, C. H. (2020). Metabolite Profiling Revealed That a Gardening Activity Program Improves Cognitive Ability Correlated with BDNF Levels and Serotonin Metabolism in the Elderly. International journal of environmental research and public health, 17(2), 541. https://doi.org/10.3390/ijerph17020541

Eco-therapy is nature's way of healing the mind: Fuller, R. A., Irvine, K. N., Devine-Wright, P., Warren, P. H., & Gaston, K. J. (2007). Psychological benefits of greenspace increase with biodiversity. Biology letters, 3(4), 390–394. https://doi.org/10.1098/rsbl.2007.0149

Biodiverse spaces bolster psychological resilience and combats urban stress: Marselle, M. R., Lindley, S. J., Cook, P. A., & Bonn, A. (2021). Biodiversity and Health in the Urban Environment. Current environmental health reports, 8(2), 146–156. https://doi.org/10.1007/s40572-021-00313-9

Methuselah: Conservation International. (2022 Jun 6). Methuselah: Still the world's oldest tree. https://www.conservation.org/blog/methuselah-still-the-worlds-oldest-tree

Wood wide web: Merckx, V. S. F. T., Gomes, S. I. F., Wang, D., Verbeek, C., Jacquemyn, H., Zahn, F. E., Gebauer, G., & Bidartondo, M. I. (2024). Mycoheterotrophy in the wood-wide web. Nature plants, 10(5), 710–718. https://doi.org/10.1038/s41477-024-01677-0

Pancha bhutas: Sadhguru. (2020). Death: An inside story: A book for all those who shall die. Penguin

Ananda.

Cold immersion offers multiple health benefits: Mohan, M. S., Sreedevi, A. S., Sakunthala, A. N., Boban, P. T., Sudhakaran, P. R., & Kamalamma, S. (2023). Intermittent cold exposure upregulates regulators of cardiac mitochondrial biogenesis and function in mice. Physiology international, 110(1), 1–18. https://doi.org/10.1556/2060.2023.00128

Cold immersion offers multiple health benefits: Srámek, P., Simecková, M., Janský, L., Savlíková, J., & Vybíral, S. (2000). Human physiological responses to immersion into water of different temperatures. European journal of applied physiology, 81(5), 436–442. https://doi.org/10.1007/s004210050065

Temperature oscillation enhances vascular tone: Moore, E., Fuller, J. T., Bellenger, C. R., Saunders, S., Halson, S. L., Broatch, J. R., & Buckley, J. D. (2023). Effects of Cold-Water Immersion Compared with Other Recovery Modalities on Athletic Performance Following Acute Strenuous Exercise in Physically Active Participants: A Systematic Review, Meta-Analysis, and Meta-Regression. Sports medicine (Auckland, N.Z.), 53(3), 687–705. https://doi.org/10.1007/s40279-022-01800-1

Cold water swimming significantly improved the mood of participants: Huttunen, P., Kokko, L., & Ylijukuri, V. (2004). Winter swimming improves general well-being. International journal of circumpolar health, 63(2), 140–144. https://doi.org/10.3402/ijch.v63i2.17700

Non-shivering thermogenesis: Klingenspor M. (2003). Cold-induced recruitment of brown adipose tissue thermogenesis. Experimental physiology, 88(1), 141–148. https://doi.org/10.1113/eph8802508

Brown adipose tissue: Lim, S., Honek, J., Xue, Y., Seki, T., Cao, Z., Andersson, P., Yang, X., Hosaka, K., & Cao, Y. (2012). Cold-induced activation of brown adipose tissue and adipose angiogenesis in mice. Nature protocols, 7(3), 606–615. https://doi.org/10.1038/nprot.2012.013

A well-synchronized circadian rhythm: Musiek, E. S., & Holtzman, D. M. (2016). Mechanisms linking circadian clocks, sleep, and neurodegeneration. Science (New York, N.Y.), 354(6315), 1004–1008. https://doi.org/10.1126/science.aah4968

Workers exposed to natural light: Boubekri, M., Cheung, I. N., Reid, K. J., Wang, C. H., & Zee, P. C. (2014). Impact of windows and daylight exposure on overall health and sleep quality of office workers: a case-control pilot study. Journal of clinical sleep medicine : JCSM : official publication of the American Academy of Sleep Medicine, 10(6), 603–611. https://doi.org/10.5664/jcsm.3780

Melatonin: Gooley, J. J., Chamberlain, K., Smith, K. A., Khalsa, S. B., Rajaratnam, S. M., Van Reen, E., Zeitzer, J. M., Czeisler, C. A., & Lockley, S. W. (2011). Exposure to room light before bedtime suppresses melatonin onset and shortens melatonin duration in humans. The Journal of clinical endocrinology and metabolism, 96(3), E463–E472. https://doi.org/10.1210/jc.2010-2098

24-hour biological cycle: Panda S. (2016). Circadian physiology of metabolism. Science (New York, N.Y.), 354(6315), 1008–1015. https://doi.org/10.1126/science.aah4967

24-hour biological cycle: Scheiermann, C., Kunisaki, Y., & Frenette, P. S. (2013). Circadian control of the immune system. Nature reviews. Immunology, 13(3), 190–198. https://doi.org/10.1038/nri3386

Biological clocks regulate gene expression: Huang R. C. (2018). The discoveries of molecular mechanisms for the circadian rhythm: The 2017 Nobel Prize in Physiology or Medicine. Biomedical journal, 41(1), 5–8. https://doi.org/10.1016/j.bj.2018.02.003

Night shift workers experience chronic inflammation: Kim SW, Jang EC, Kwon SC, Han W, Kang MS, Nam YH, Lee YJ. Night shift work and inflammatory markers in male workers aged 20-39 in a display manufacturing company. Ann Occup Environ Med. 2016 Sep 20;28:48. doi: 10.1186/s40557-016-0135-y. PMID: 27660715; PMCID: PMC5028985.

Recalibrating your circadian rhythm: Wright, K. P., Jr, McHill, A. W., Birks, B. R., Griffin, B. R., Rusterholz, T., & Chinoy, E. D. (2013). Entrainment of the human circadian clock to the natural light-dark cycle. Current biology : CB, 23(16), 1554–1558. https://doi.org/10.1016/j.cub.2013.06.039

Chapter 2

Elevated VO2 max levels are associated with lower risks of cardiovascular diseases: Kodama, S., Saito, K., Tanaka, S., Maki, M., Yachi, Y., Asumi, M., Sugawara, A., Totsuka, K., Shimano, H., Ohashi, Y., Yamada, N., & Sone, H. (2009). Cardiorespiratory fitness as a quantitative predictor of all-cause mortality and cardiovascular events in healthy men and women: a meta-analysis. JAMA, 301(19), 2024–2035. https://doi.org/10.1001/jama.2009.681

Greater muscle strength is linked to a lower risk of all-cause mortality: García-Hermoso, A., Cavero-Redondo, I., Ramírez-Vélez, R., Ruiz, J. R., Ortega, F. B., Lee, D. C., & Martínez-Vizcaíno, V. (2018). Muscular Strength as a Predictor of All-Cause Mortality in an Apparently Healthy Population: A Systematic Review and Meta-Analysis of Data From Approximately 2 Million Men and Women. Archives of physical medicine and rehabilitation, 99(10), 2100–2113.e5. https://doi.org/10.1016/j.apmr.2018.01.008

Muscle strength: Westcott WL. Resistance training is medicine: effects of strength training on health. Curr Sports Med Rep. 2012 Jul-Aug;11(4):209-16. doi: 10.1249/JSR.0b013e31825dabb8. PMID: 22777332.

Squatting: Schoenfeld BJ. Squatting kinematics and kinetics and their application to exercise performance. J Strength Cond Res. 2010 Dec;24(12):3497-506. doi: 10.1519/JSC.0b013e3181bac2d7. PMID: 20182386.

Proper posture: Toprak Çelenay, Ş., & Özer Kaya, D. (2017). An 8-week thoracic spine stabilization exercise program improves postural back pain, spine alignment, postural sway, and core endurance in university students:a randomized controlled study. Turkish journal of medical sciences, 47(2), 504–513. https://doi.org/10.3906/sag-1511-155

Posture: Korakakis, V., O'Sullivan, K., O'Sullivan, P. B., Evagelinou, V., Sotiralis, Y., Sideris, A., Sakellariou, K., Karanasios, S., & Giakas, G. (2019). Physiotherapist perceptions of optimal sitting and standing posture. Musculoskeletal science & practice, 39, 24–31. https://doi.org/10.1016/j.msksp.2018.11.004

Lumbar spine: McGill, S. (2007). Low back disorders: Evidence-based prevention and rehabilitation (2nd ed.). Human Kinetics.

Sitting is the new smoking: Starrett, K., Starrett, J., & Cordoza, G. (2016). Deskbound: Standing up to a sitting world. Victory Belt Publishing.

Prolonged sitting can lead to a series of adverse health effects: Patel, A. V., Maliniak, M. L., Rees-

Punia, E., Matthews, C. E., & Gapstur, S. M. (2018). Prolonged Leisure Time Spent Sitting in Relation to Cause-Specific Mortality in a Large US Cohort. American journal of epidemiology, 187(10), 2151–2158. https://doi.org/10.1093/aje/kwy125

Prolonged sitting: Owen, N., Healy, G. N., Matthews, C. E., & Dunstan, D. W. (2010). Too much sitting: the population health science of sedentary behavior. Exercise and sport sciences reviews, 38(3), 105–113. https://doi.org/10.1097/JES.0b013e3181e373a2

Prolonged sitting: Edwardson, C. L., Biddle, S. J. H., Clemes, S. A., Davies, M. J., Dunstan, D. W., Eborall, H., Granat, M. H., Gray, L. J., Healy, G. N., Jaicim, N. B., Lawton, S., Maylor, B. D., Munir, F., Richardson, G., Yates, T., & Clarke-Cornwell, A. M. (2022). Effectiveness of an intervention for reducing sitting time and improving health in office workers: three arm cluster randomised controlled trial. BMJ (Clinical research ed.), 378, e069288. https://doi.org/10.1136/bmj-2021-069288

Prolonged sitting: Baker, R., Coenen, P., Howie, E., Williamson, A., & Straker, L. (2018). The Short Term Musculoskeletal and Cognitive Effects of Prolonged Sitting During Office Computer Work. International journal of environmental research and public health, 15(8), 1678. https://doi.org/10.3390/ijerph15081678

Dormant butt syndrome: Kolba, C. (2023, January 12). Knee, hip or back pain? dormant butt syndrome may be to blame. Ohio State Health and Discovery. https://health.osu.edu/health/bone-and-joint/dormant-butt-syndrome-and-joint-pain

Desk Ergonomics: Lee, S., DE Barros, F. C., DE Castro, C. S. M., & DE Oliveira Sato, T. (2021). Effect of an ergonomic intervention involving workstation adjustments on musculoskeletal pain in office workers-a randomized controlled clinical trial. Industrial health, 59(2), 78–85. https://doi.org/10.2486/indhealth.2020-0188

Forward head posture: Sheikhhoseini, R., Shahrbanian, S., Sayyadi, P., & O'Sullivan, K. (2018). Effectiveness of Therapeutic Exercise on Forward Head Posture: A Systematic Review and Meta-analysis. Journal of manipulative and physiological therapeutics, 41(6), 530–539. https://doi.org/10.1016/j.jmpt.2018.02.002.

Forward head posture: Sepehri, S., Sheikhhoseini, R., Piri, H., & Sayyadi, P. (2024). The effect of various therapeutic exercises on forward head posture, rounded shoulder, and hyperkyphosis among people with upper crossed syndrome: a systematic review and meta-analysis. BMC musculoskeletal disorders, 25(1), 105. https://doi.org/10.1186/s12891-024-07224-4

Tension myositis syndrome: Sarno J. E. (1977). Psychosomatic backache. The Journal of family practice, 5(3), 353–357.

Tension myositis syndrome: Schechter, D., Smith, A. P., Beck, J., Roach, J., Karim, R., & Azen, S. (2007). Outcomes of a mind-body treatment program for chronic back pain with no distinct structural pathology--a case series of patients diagnosed and treated as tension myositis syndrome. Alternative therapies in health and medicine, 13(5), 26–35.

Trigger points: Money S. (2017). Pathophysiology of Trigger Points in Myofascial Pain Syndrome. Journal of pain & palliative care pharmacotherapy, 31(2), 158–159. https://doi.org/10.1080/15360288.2017.1298688

Trigger points, targeted release: Lew, J., Kim, J., & Nair, P. (2021). Comparison of dry needling and trigger point manual therapy in patients with neck and upper back myofascial pain syndrome: a systematic review and meta-analysis. The Journal of manual & manipulative therapy, 29(3), 136–146. https://doi.org/10.1080/10669817.2020.1822618

Shoulder function: Veeger, H. E., & van der Helm, F. C. (2007). Shoulder function: the perfect compromise between mobility and stability. Journal of biomechanics, 40(10), 2119–2129. https://doi.org/10.1016/j.jbiomech.2006.10.016

Shoulder impingement: Lewis J. S. (2010). Rotator cuff tendinopathy: a model for the continuum of pathology and related management. British journal of sports medicine, 44(13), 918–923. https://doi.org/10.1136/bjsm.2008.054817

Diagnostic imaging of shoulder: Seeger, L. L., Gold, R. H., Bassett, L. W., & Ellman, H. (1988). Shoulder impingement syndrome: MR findings in 53 shoulders. AJR. American journal of roentgenology, 150(2), 343–347. https://doi.org/10.2214/ajr.150.2.343

Functional movement: Cook, G. (2010). Movement: Functional movement systems: Screening, assessment, and corrective strategies. On Target Publications.

Exercises that replicate real-life movements can boost functionality and reduce injury risk: Koźlenia, D., & Domaradzki, J. (2021). Prediction and injury risk based on movement patterns and flexibility in a 6-month prospective study among physically active adults. PeerJ, 9, e11399. https://doi.org/10.7717/peerj.11399

Functional exercises: Buxton, J. D., Prins, P. J., Miller, M. G., Moreno, A., Welton, G. L., Atwell, A. D., Talampas, T. R., & Elsey, G. E. (2022). The Effects of a Novel Quadrupedal Movement Training Program on Functional Movement, Range of Motion, Muscular Strength, and Endurance. Journal of strength and conditioning research, 36(8), 2186–2193. https://doi.org/10.1519/JSC.0000000000003818

Functional movements, mind-body connection: Wills, J. A., Saxby, D. J., Glassbrook, D. J., & Doyle, T. L. A. (2019). Load-Carriage Conditioning Elicits Task-Specific Physical and Psychophysical Improvements in Males. Journal of strength and conditioning research, 33(9), 2338–2343. https://doi.org/10.1519/JSC.0000000000003243

Rucking: Earl-Boehm, J. E., Poel, D. N., Zalewski, K., & Ebersole, K. T. (2020). The effects of military style ruck marching on lower extremity loading and muscular, physiological and perceived exertion in ROTC cadets. Ergonomics, 63(5), 629–638. https://doi.org/10.1080/00140139.2020.1745900

Rucking can burn significant calories: Quesada, P. M., Mengelkoch, L. J., Hale, R. C., & Simon, S. R. (2000). Biomechanical and metabolic effects of varying backpack loading on simulated marching. Ergonomics, 43(3), 293–309. https://doi.org/10.1080/001401300184413

Norwegian protocol: Wisløff, U., Nilsen, T. I., Drøyvold, W. B., Mørkved, S., Slørdahl, S. A., & Vatten, L. J. (2006). A single weekly bout of exercise may reduce cardiovascular mortality: how little pain for cardiac gain? 'The HUNT study, Norway'. European journal of cardiovascular prevention and rehabilitation : official journal of the European Society of Cardiology, Working Groups on Epidemiology & Prevention and Cardiac Rehabilitation and Exercise Physiology, 13(5), 798–804. https://doi.org/10.1097/01.hjr.0000216548.84560.ac

High-Intensity Interval Training (HIIT): Helgerud, J., Høydal, K., Wang, E., Karlsen, T., Berg, P., Bjerkaas, M., Simonsen, T., Helgesen, C., Hjorth, N., Bach, R., & Hoff, J. (2007). Aerobic high-intensity intervals improve VO2max more than moderate training. Medicine and science in sports and exercise, 39(4), 665–671. https://doi.org/10.1249/mss.0b013e3180304570

Controlled articular rotations: Gharisia, O., Lohman, E., Daher, N., Eldridge, A., Shallan, A., & Jaber, H. (2021). Effect of a novel stretching technique on shoulder range of motion in overhead athletes with glenohumeral internal rotation deficits: a randomized controlled trial. BMC musculoskeletal disorders, 22(1), 402. https://doi.org/10.1186/s12891-021-04292-8

Human skulls have evolved: Evensen, J. P., & Øgaard, B. (2007). Are malocclusions more prevalent and severe now? A comparative study of medieval skulls from Norway. American journal of orthodontics and dentofacial orthopedics : official publication of the American Association of Orthodontists, its constituent societies, and the American Board of Orthodontics, 131(6), 710–716. https://doi.org/10.1016/j.ajodo.2005.08.037

Skull shape and size: Sambataro, S., Fiorillo, L., Bocchieri, S., Stumpo, C., Cervino, G., Herford, A. S., & Cicciù, M. (2022). Craniofacial Evolution: From Australopithecus to Modern Man. The Journal of craniofacial surgery, 33(1), 325–332. https://doi.org/10.1097/SCS.0000000000007841

Jaw and dental arch: Boyd, K. L., Saccomanno, S., Coceani Paskay Hv, L., Quinzi, V., & Marzo, G. (2021). Maldevelopment of the cranio-facial-respiratory complex: A Darwinian perspective. European journal of paediatric dentistry, 22(3), 225–229. https://doi.org/10.23804/ejpd.2021.22.03.9

Breathing patterns: Fagundes, N. C. F., Gianoni-Capenakas, S., Heo, G., & Flores-Mir, C. (2022). Craniofacial features in children with obstructive sleep apnea: a systematic review and meta-analysis. Journal of clinical sleep medicine : JCSM : official publication of the American Academy of Sleep Medicine, 18(7), 1865–1875. https://doi.org/10.5664/jcsm.9904

Obstructive sleep apnea: Neelapu BC, Kharbanda OP, Sardana HK, Balachandran R, Sardana V, Kapoor P, Gupta A, Vasamsetti S. Craniofacial and upper airway morphology in adult obstructive sleep apnea patients: A systematic review and meta-analysis of cephalometric studies. Sleep Med Rev. 2017 Feb;31:79-90. doi: 10.1016/j.smrv.2016.01.007. Epub 2016 Jan 30. PMID: 27039222.

Dental arch reduction: Irlandese, G., De Stefani, A., Mezzofranco, L., Milano, F., Di Giosia, M., Bruno, G., & Gracco, A. (2023). Dental arch form and interdental widths evaluation in adult Caucasian patients with obstructive sleep apnea syndrome. Cranio : the journal of craniomandibular practice, 41(2), 151–159. https://doi.org/10.1080/08869634.2020.1802949

Tai Chi, mental clarity: Wayne, P. M., Walsh, J. N., Taylor-Piliae, R. E., Wells, R. E., Papp, K. V., Donovan, N. J., & Yeh, G. Y. (2014). Effect of tai chi on cognitive performance in older adults: systematic review and meta-analysis. Journal of the American Geriatrics Society, 62(1), 25–39. https://doi.org/10.1111/jgs.12611

Tai Chi reduces falls in older adults: Low, S., Ang, L. W., Goh, K. S., & Chew, S. K. (2009). A systematic review of the effectiveness of Tai Chi on fall reduction among the elderly. Archives of gerontology and geriatrics, 48(3), 325–331. https://doi.org/10.1016/j.archger.2008.02.018

Proprioception: Rivera, M. J., Winkelmann, Z. K., Powden, C. J., & Games, K. E. (2017). Proprioceptive Training for the Prevention of Ankle Sprains: An Evidence-Based Review. Journal of athletic training, 52(11), 1065–1067. https://doi.org/10.4085/1062-6050-52.11.16

Interoception: Critchley, H. D., Wiens, S., Rotshtein, P., Ohman, A., & Dolan, R. J. (2004). Neural systems supporting interoceptive awareness. Nature neuroscience, 7(2), 189–195. https://doi.org/10.1038/nn1176

Chapter 3

Hadzabe's dietary patterns: Marlowe, F. W., & Berbesque, J. C. (2009). Tubers as fallback foods and their impact on Hadza hunter-gatherers. American journal of physical anthropology, 140(4), 751–758. https://doi.org/10.1002/ajpa.21040

Hadzabe's dietary patterns: Pontzer, H., & Wood, B. M. (2021). Effects of Evolution, Ecology, and Economy on Human Diet: Insights from Hunter-Gatherers and Other Small-Scale Societies. Annual review of nutrition, 41, 363–385. https://doi.org/10.1146/annurev-nutr-111120-105520

Hadzabe, active lifestyle: Sayre, M. K., Pontzer, H., Alexander, G. E., Wood, B. M., Pike, I. L., Mabulla, A. Z. P., & Raichlen, D. A. (2020). Ageing and physical function in East African foragers and pastoralists. Philosophical transactions of the Royal Society of London. Series B, Biological sciences, 375(1811), 20190608. https://doi.org/10.1098/rstb.2019.0608

Hadzabe, cardiovascular health: Raichlen, D. A., Pontzer, H., Harris, J. A., Mabulla, A. Z., Marlowe, F. W., Josh Snodgrass, J., Eick, G., Colette Berbesque, J., Sancilio, A., & Wood, B. M. (2017). Physical activity patterns and biomarkers of cardiovascular disease risk in hunter-gatherers. American journal of human biology : the official journal of the Human Biology Council, 29(2), 10.1002/ajhb.22919. https://doi.org/10.1002/ajhb.22919

Intermittent fasting (IF) and time-restricted eating: Longo, V. D., & Panda, S. (2016). Fasting, Circadian Rhythms, and Time-Restricted Feeding in Healthy Lifespan. Cell metabolism, 23(6), 1048–1059. https://doi.org/10.1016/j.cmet.2016.06.001

Intermittent fasting: de Cabo, R., & Mattson, M. P. (2019). Effects of Intermittent Fasting on Health, Aging, and Disease. The New England journal of medicine, 381(26), 2541–2551. https://doi.org/10.1056/NEJMra1905136

Fasting triggers autophagy: Liu, S., Zeng, M., Wan, W., Huang, M., Li, X., Xie, Z., Wang, S., & Cai, Y. (2023). The Health-Promoting Effects and the Mechanism of Intermittent Fasting. Journal of diabetes research, 2023, 4038546. https://doi.org/10.1155/2023/4038546

Intermittent fasting can significantly improve insulin sensitivity: Sutton, E. F., Beyl, R., Early, K. S., Cefalu, W. T., Ravussin, E., & Peterson, C. M. (2018). Early Time-Restricted Feeding Improves Insulin Sensitivity, Blood Pressure, and Oxidative Stress Even without Weight Loss in Men with Prediabetes. Cell metabolism, 27(6), 1212–1221.e3. https://doi.org/10.1016/j.cmet.2018.04.010

Intermittent fasting has been linked to neuroprotection: Mattson, M. P., Moehl, K., Ghena, N., Schmaedick, M., & Cheng, A. (2018). Intermittent metabolic switching, neuroplasticity and brain health. Nature reviews. Neuroscience, 19(2), 63–80. https://doi.org/10.1038/nrn.2017.156

Gut microbiome is like a unique fingerprint shaped by genetics, diet, and lifestyle: David, L. A., Maurice, C. F., Carmody, R. N., Gootenberg, D. B., Button, J. E., Wolfe, B. E., Ling, A. V., Devlin, A. S., Varma, Y., Fischbach, M. A., Biddinger, S. B., Dutton, R. J., & Turnbaugh, P. J. (2014). Diet rapidly and reproducibly alters the human gut microbiome. Nature, 505(7484), 559–563. https://doi.org/10.1038/nature12820

Greater microbial diversity correlates with better health outcomes: Badal, V. D., Vaccariello, E. D., Murray, E. R., Yu, K. E., Knight, R., Jeste, D. V., & Nguyen, T. T. (2020). The Gut Microbiome, Aging, and Longevity: A Systematic Review. Nutrients, 12(12), 3759. https://doi.org/10.3390/nu12123759

Short-chain fatty acids (SCFAs): Martin-Gallausiaux, C., Marinelli, L., Blottière, H. M., Larraufie, P., & Lapaque, N. (2021). SCFA: mechanisms and functional importance in the gut. The Proceedings of the Nutrition Society, 80(1), 37–49. https://doi.org/10.1017/S0029665120006916

Gut, a pivotal player in immune response: Shi N, Li N, Duan X, Niu H. Interaction between the gut microbiome and mucosal immune system. Mil Med Res. 2017 Apr 27;4:14. doi: 10.1186/s40779-017-0122-9. PMID: 28465831; PMCID: PMC5408367.

Gut and brain are constantly conversing: Osadchiy, V., Martin, C. R., & Mayer, E. A. (2019). The Gut-Brain Axis and the Microbiome: Mechanisms and Clinical Implications. Clinical gastroenterology and hepatology : the official clinical practice journal of the American Gastroenterological Association, 17(2), 322–332. https://doi.org/10.1016/j.cgh.2018.10.002

Some gut bacteria generate serotonin: O'Mahony, S. M., Clarke, G., Borre, Y. E., Dinan, T. G., & Cryan, J. F. (2015). Serotonin, tryptophan metabolism and the brain-gut-microbiome axis. Behavioural brain research, 277, 32–48. https://doi.org/10.1016/j.bbr.2014.07.027

Healthy gut ecosystems: Manos J. (2022). The human microbiome in disease and pathology. APMIS : acta pathologica, microbiologica, et immunologica Scandinavica, 130(12), 690–705. https://doi.org/10.1111/apm.13225

Prebiotic fibers, microbial diversity: Sonnenburg, E. D., Smits, S. A., Tikhonov, M., Higginbottom, S. K., Wingreen, N. S., & Sonnenburg, J. L. (2016). Diet-induced extinctions in the gut microbiota compound over generations. Nature, 529(7585), 212–215. https://doi.org/10.1038/nature16504

Diet, microbial diversity: De Filippo, C., Cavalieri, D., Di Paola, M., Ramazzotti, M., Poullet, J. B., Massart, S., Collini, S., Pieraccini, G., & Lionetti, P. (2010). Impact of diet in shaping gut microbiota revealed by a comparative study in children from Europe and rural Africa. Proceedings of the National Academy of Sciences of the United States of America, 107(33), 14691–14696. https://doi.org/10.1073/pnas.1005963107

Consuming fresh produce from the season: Macdiarmid J. I. (2014). Seasonality and dietary requirements: will eating seasonal food contribute to health and environmental sustainability?. The Proceedings of the Nutrition Society, 73(3), 368–375. https://doi.org/10.1017/S0029665113003753

Psychological benefits of mindfulness in eating: Kristeller, J. L., & Wolever, R. Q. (2011). Mindfulness-based eating awareness training for treating binge eating disorder: the conceptual foundation. Eating disorders, 19(1), 49–61. https://doi.org/10.1080/10640266.2011.533605

Modern diets rich in such calorie-dense and nutrient-poor foods: Monteiro, C. A., Cannon, G., Levy, R. B., Moubarac, J. C., Louzada, M. L., Rauber, F., Khandpur, N., Cediel, G., Neri, D., Martinez-Steele, E., Baraldi, L. G., & Jaime, P. C. (2019). Ultra-processed foods: what they are and how to identify them. Public health nutrition, 22(5), 936–941. https://doi.org/10.1017/S1368980018003762

Nutrient density: Drewnowski, A., & Fulgoni, V., 3rd (2008). Nutrient profiling of foods: creating a nutrient-rich food index. Nutrition reviews, 66(1), 23–39. https://doi.org/10.1111/j.1753-4887.2007.00003.x

Soil depletion: Soil erosion. (2023, June 7). Undrr.org. https://www.undrr.org/understanding-disaster-risk/terminology/hips/en0019

Soil nutrient depletion: European Commission: Joint Research Centre, Hill, J., Von Maltitz, G.,

Sommer, S., Reynolds, J., Hutchinson, C., & Cherlet, M. (2018). World atlas of desertification : rethinking land degradation and sustainable land management, (J.Hill,editor,G.Von Maltitz,editor,S. Sommer,editor,J.Reynolds,editor,C.Hutchinson,editor,M.Cherlet,edito) Publications Office. https:// data.europa.eu/doi/10.2760/06292

Crop nutrient levels can significantly vary based on soil health and farming practices: Tiong, Y. W., Sharma, P., Xu, S., Bu, J., An, S., Foo, J. B. L., Wee, B. K., Wang, Y., Lee, J. T. E., Zhang, J., He, Y., & Tong, Y. W. (2024). Enhancing sustainable crop cultivation: The impact of renewable soil amendments and digestate fertilizer on crop growth and nutrient composition. Environmental pollution (Barking, Essex : 1987), 342, 123132. https://doi.org/10.1016/j.envpol.2023.123132

Crop nutrient levels can significantly vary based on soil health and farming practices: Montgomery, D. R., Biklé, A., Archuleta, R., Brown, P., & Jordan, J. (2022). Soil health and nutrient density: preliminary comparison of regenerative and conventional farming. PeerJ, 10, e12848. https://doi. org/10.7717/peerj.12848

Backing regenerative agriculture fosters healthier ecosystems that produce nutrient-dense foods: Manzeke-Kangara, M. G., Joy, E. J. M., Lark, R. M., Redfern, S., Eilander, A., & Broadley, M. R. (2023). Do agronomic approaches aligned to regenerative agriculture improve the micronutrient concentrations of edible portions of crops? A scoping review of evidence. Frontiers in nutrition, 10, 1078667. https://doi.org/10.3389/fnut.2023.1078667

Mitochondrial biogenesis: Hood, D. A., Uguccioni, G., Vainshtein, A., & D'souza, D. (2011). Mechanisms of exercise-induced mitochondrial biogenesis in skeletal muscle: implications for health and disease. Comprehensive Physiology, 1(3), 1119–1134. https://doi.org/10.1002/cphy.c100074

Mitochondrial dynamics: Westermann B. (2012). Bioenergetic role of mitochondrial fusion and fission. Biochimica et biophysica acta, 1817(10), 1833–1838. https://doi.org/10.1016/j.bbabio.2012.02.033

Mitophagy: Liu, B. H., Xu, C. Z., Liu, Y., Lu, Z. L., Fu, T. L., Li, G. R., Deng, Y., Luo, G. Q., Ding, S., Li, N., & Geng, Q. (2024). Mitochondrial quality control in human health and disease. Military Medical Research, 11(1), 32. https://doi.org/10.1186/s40779-024-00536-5

Average American consumes about 17 teaspoons of added sugar per day: Powell, J. (2013, August 5). Added sugar. The Nutrition Source. https://nutritionsource.hsph.harvard.edu/carbohydrates/ added-sugar-in-the-diet/

Sugars, metabolic dysfuntion: Ludwig D. S. (2002). The glycemic index: physiological mechanisms relating to obesity, diabetes, and cardiovascular disease. JAMA, 287(18), 2414–2423. https://doi. org/10.1001/jama.287.18.2414

Sugars, cardiovascular health: Johnson, R. K., Appel, L. J., Brands, M., Howard, B. V., Lefevre, M., Lustig, R. H., Sacks, F., Steffen, L. M., Wylie-Rosett, J., & American Heart Association Nutrition Committee of the Council on Nutrition, Physical Activity, and Metabolism and the Council on Epidemiology and Prevention (2009). Dietary sugars intake and cardiovascular health: a scientific statement from the American Heart Association. Circulation, 120(11), 1011–1020. https://doi. org/10.1161/CIRCULATIONAHA.109.192627

Epigenetics and nutrition: Environment and epigenetics: Feil, R., & Fraga, M. F. (2012). Epigenetics and the environment: emerging patterns and implications. Nature reviews. Genetics, 13(2), 97–109. https://doi.org/10.1038/nrg3142

Diet can activate or silence genes through DNA methylation and histone modification: Mierziak, J., Kostyn, K., Boba, A., Czemplik, M., Kulma, A., & Wojtasik, W. (2021). Influence of the Bioactive Diet Components on the Gene Expression Regulation. Nutrients, 13(11), 3673. https://doi.org/10.3390/nu13113673

Sattvic, Rajasic, and Tamasic categories: Gerson, S. (2002). The Ayurvedic guide to diet. Lotus Press. ISBN 978-0-910261-29-6.

Chapter 4

Chitta Vritti Nirodhah: Patanjali. (2001). The Yoga Sutras of Patanjali (E. Bryant, Trans.). North Point Press. (Original work published ca. 400 CE)

Stress has an evolutionary origin: Davidson, R. J., & McEwen, B. S. (2012). Social influences on neuroplasticity: stress and interventions to promote well-being. Nature neuroscience, 15(5), 689–695. https://doi.org/10.1038/nn.3093

Stress has an evolutionary origin: McEwen B. S. (2007). Physiology and neurobiology of stress and adaptation: central role of the brain. Physiological reviews, 87(3), 873–904. https://doi.org/10.1152/physrev.00041.2006

Telomere shortening: Effros R. B. (2011). Telomere/telomerase dynamics within the human immune system: effect of chronic infection and stress. Experimental gerontology, 46(2-3), 135–140. https://doi.org/10.1016/j.exger.2010.08.027

Telomere shortening: Biegler, K. A., Anderson, A. K., Wenzel, L. B., Osann, K., & Nelson, E. L. (2012). Longitudinal change in telomere length and the chronic stress response in a randomized pilot biobehavioral clinical study: implications for cancer prevention. Cancer prevention research (Philadelphia, Pa.), 5(10), 1173–1182. https://doi.org/10.1158/1940-6207.CAPR-12-0008

Neuroplasticity: Merzenich, M. M. (2009). Soft-wired: How the new science of brain plasticity can change your life. Parnassus Publishing.

Neuroplasticity: Kramer AF, Bherer L, Colcombe SJ, Dong W, Greenough WT. Environmental influences on cognitive and brain plasticity during aging. J Gerontol A Biol Sci Med Sci. 2004 Sep;59(9):M940-57. doi: 10.1093/gerona/59.9.m940. PMID: 15472160.

Mindfulness meditation increased cortical thickness: Lazar SW, Kerr CE, Wasserman RH, Gray JR, Greve DN, Treadway MT, McGarvey M, Quinn BT, Dusek JA, Benson H, Rauch SL, Moore CI, Fischl B. Meditation experience is associated with increased cortical thickness. Neuroreport. 2005 Nov 28;16(17):1893-7. doi: 10.1097/01.wnr.0000186598.66243.19. PMID: 16272874; PMCID: PMC1361002.

Long-term meditators who demonstrated brains remarkably younger: Luders, E., Kurth, F., Mayer, E. A., Toga, A. W., Narr, K. L., & Gaser, C. (2012). The unique brain anatomy of meditation practitioners: alterations in cortical gyrification. Frontiers in human neuroscience, 6, 34. https://doi.org/10.3389/fnhum.2012.00034

Brain energy demands: Raichle, M. E., & Gusnard, D. A. (2002). Appraising the brain's energy budget. Proceedings of the National Academy of Sciences of the United States of America, 99(16), 10237–10239. https://doi.org/10.1073/pnas.172399499

Anapanasati yoga: Bodhi, B. (Trans.). (2000). The connected discourses of the Buddha: A new translation of the Saṃyutta Nikāya (Vol. 2). Wisdom Publications. (Original work ca. 5th century BCE – Ānāpānasati Sutta appears in Majjhima Nikāya 118 and Saṃyutta Nikāya 54)

Breathing-focused practices have been linked to reduced stress levels, improved emotional regulation: Brown, R. P., & Gerbarg, P. L. (2005). Sudarshan Kriya yogic breathing in the treatment of stress, anxiety, and depression: part I-neurophysiologic model. Journal of alternative and complementary medicine (New York, N.Y.), 11(1), 189–201. https://doi.org/10.1089/acm.2005.11.189

Wandering mind: Cohen, M. R., & Maunsell, J. H. (2011). When attention wanders: how uncontrolled fluctuations in attention affect performance. The Journal of neuroscience : the official journal of the Society for Neuroscience, 31(44), 15802–15806. https://doi.org/10.1523/JNEUROSCI.3063-11.2011

Default Mode Network (DMN): Zagkas, D., Bacopoulou, F., Vlachakis, D., Chrousos, G. P., & Darviri, C. (2023). How Does Meditation Affect the Default Mode Network: A Systematic Review. Advances in experimental medicine and biology, 1425, 229–245. https://doi.org/10.1007/978-3-031-31986-0_22

The slower we breathe, the slower our metabolic rate: Zaccaro, A., Piarulli, A., Laurino, M., Garbella, E., Menicucci, D., Neri, B., & Gemignani, A. (2018). How Breath-Control Can Change Your Life: A Systematic Review on Psycho-Physiological Correlates of Slow Breathing. Frontiers in human neuroscience, 12, 353. https://doi.org/10.3389/fnhum.2018.00353

Pranayama is a powerful longevity tool: Kumar, S. B., Yadav, R., Yadav, R. K., Tolahunase, M., & Dada, R. (2015). Telomerase activity and cellular aging might be positively modified by a yoga-based lifestyle intervention. Journal of alternative and complementary medicine (New York, N.Y.), 21(6), 370–372. https://doi.org/10.1089/acm.2014.0298

Pranayama is a powerful longevity tool: Mony, V., Subramanian, S., & Kanchibhotla, D. (2025). Sudarshan Kriya Yoga Promotes Telomere Elongation: A Pilot Study. Alternative therapies in health and medicine, 31(2), 6–11.

Pranayama is a powerful longevity tool: Rathore, M., & Abraham, J. (2018). Implication of Asana, Pranayama and Meditation on Telomere Stability. International journal of yoga, 11(3), 186–193. https://doi.org/10.4103/ijoy.IJOY_51_17

Pranayama, oxygen efficiency: Campanelli, S., Lopes Tort, A. B., & Lobão-Soares, B. (2020). Pranayamas and Their Neurophysiological Effects. International Journal of Yoga, 13(3), 183. https://doi.org/10.4103/ijoy.IJOY_91_19

Higher CO_2 tolerance: Porcari, J. P., Probst, L., Forrester, K., Doberstein, S., Foster, C., Cress, M. L., & Schmidt, K. (2016). Effect of Wearing the Elevation Training Mask on Aerobic Capacity, Lung Function, and Hematological Variables. Journal of Sports Science & Medicine, 15(2), 379. https://pmc.ncbi.nlm.nih.gov/articles/PMC4879455/

Second brain: Gershon, M. D. (1998). The Second Brain: Your Gut Has a Mind of Its Own. HarperCollins.

Gut-brain axis: Cryan, J. F., & Dinan, T. G. (2012). Mind-altering microorganisms: the impact of the gut microbiota on brain and behaviour. Nature reviews. Neuroscience, 13(10), 701–712. https://doi.

org/10.1038/nrn3346

Gut-brain axis: Sampson, T. R., & Mazmanian, S. K. (2015). Control of brain development, function, and behavior by the microbiome. Cell host & microbe, 17(5), 565–576. https://doi.org/10.1016/j.chom.2015.04.011

Gut-brain axis: Mayer E. A. (2011). Gut feelings: the emerging biology of gut-brain communication. Nature reviews. Neuroscience, 12(8), 453–466. https://doi.org/10.1038/nrn3071

Heart-brain dialogue: Alshami A. M. (2019). Pain: Is It All in the Brain or the Heart?. Current pain and headache reports, 23(12), 88. https://doi.org/10.1007/s11916-019-0827-4

Heart coherence: McCraty R, Atkinson M, Tomasino D, Bradley RT (n.d.). Coherent heart: Heart-Brain Interactions, Psychophysiological Coherence, and the Emergence of system-Wide Order. HeartMath Institute. Retrieved April 5, 2025, from https://www.heartmath.org/resources/downloads/coherent-heart/

MRI studies have shown that regular yoga can increase gray matter in brain regions related to stress regulation: Kral, T. R. A., Schuyler, B. S., Mumford, J. A., Rosenkranz, M. A., Lutz, A., & Davidson, R. J. (2018). Impact of short- and long-term mindfulness meditation training on amygdala reactivity to emotional stimuli. NeuroImage, 181, 301–313. https://doi.org/10.1016/j.neuroimage.2018.07.013

Yoga enhances proprioception: Cherup, N. P., Strand, K. L., Lucchi, L., Wooten, S. V., Luca, C., & Signorile, J. F. (2021). Yoga Meditation Enhances Proprioception and Balance in Individuals Diagnosed With Parkinson's Disease. Perceptual and motor skills, 128(1), 304–323. https://doi.org/10.1177/0031512520945085

Insufficient sleep is associated with a higher mortality risk: Cappuccio, F. P., D'Elia, L., Strazzullo, P., & Miller, M. A. (2010). Sleep duration and all-cause mortality: a systematic review and meta-analysis of prospective studies. Sleep, 33(5), 585–592. https://doi.org/10.1093/sleep/33.5.585

But why is sleep so important for our brain's well-being?: Walker, M. (2017) Why We Sleep: Unlocking the Power of Sleep and Dreams. Scribner, New York.

Deep sleep, biological necessity: Irwin M. R. (2015). Why sleep is important for health: a psychoneuroimmunology perspective. Annual review of psychology, 66, 143–172. https://doi.org/10.1146/annurev-psych-010213-115205

Brain detoxifies, beta-amyloid: Xie, L., Kang, H., Xu, Q., Chen, M. J., Liao, Y., Thiyagarajan, M., O'Donnell, J., Christensen, D. J., Nicholson, C., Iliff, J. J., Takano, T., Deane, R., & Nedergaard, M. (2013). Sleep drives metabolite clearance from the adult brain. Science (New York, N.Y.), 342(6156), 373–377. https://doi.org/10.1126/science.1241224

Artificial light confusion: Wright, K. P., Jr, McHill, A. W., Birks, B. R., Griffin, B. R., Rusterholz, T., & Chinoy, E. D. (2013). Entrainment of the human circadian clock to the natural light-dark cycle. Current biology : CB, 23(16), 1554–1558. https://doi.org/10.1016/j.cub.2013.06.039

Sleep and sunlight: Anderson, A. R., Ostermiller, L., Lastrapes, M., & Hales, L. (2024). Does sunlight exposure predict next-night sleep? A daily diary study among U.S. adults. Journal of health psychology, 13591053241262643. Advance online publication. https://doi.org/10.1177/13591053241262643

Caffeine: Gardiner, C., Weakley, J., Burke, L. M., Roach, G. D., Sargent, C., Maniar, N., Townshend,

A., & Halson, S. L. (2023). The effect of caffeine on subsequent sleep: A systematic review and meta-analysis. Sleep medicine reviews, 69, 101764. https://doi.org/10.1016/j.smrv.2023.101764

Deep work: Newport, C. (2016). Deep work: Rules for focused success in a distracted world. Grand Central Publishing.

Sat Chit Anand: Yogananda, P. (2005). Autobiography of a Yogi (Reprint ed.). Self-Realization Fellowship. (Original work published 1946)

Chapter 5

Purposeful actions, dopamine: Westbrook, A., van den Bosch, R., Määttä, J. I., Hofmans, L., Papadopetraki, D., Cools, R., & Frank, M. J. (2020). Dopamine promotes cognitive effort by biasing the benefits versus costs of cognitive work. Science (New York, N.Y.), 367(6484), 1362–1366. https://doi.org/10.1126/science.aaz5891

Victor Frankl: Frankl, V. E. (2006). Man's search for meaning (I. Lasch, Trans.). Beacon Press. (Original work published 1946)

Finding your ikigai: García, H., & Miralles, F. (2017). Ikigai: The Japanese secret to a long and happy life (H. Salazar, Trans.). Penguin Books.

Flow state: Abuhamdeh S. (2020). Investigating the "Flow" Experience: Key Conceptual and Operational Issues. Frontiers in psychology, 11, 158. https://doi.org/10.3389/fpsyg.2020.00158

Mihaly Csikszentmihalyi: Csikszentmihalyi, M., & Lebuda, I. (2017). A Window Into the Bright Side of Psychology: Interview With Mihaly Csikszentmihalyi. Europe's journal of psychology, 13(4), 810–821. https://doi.org/10.5964/ejop.v13i4.1482

Flow state, functional MRI: Ulrich, M., Keller, J., & Grön, G. (2015). Neural signatures of experimentally induced flow experiences identified in a typical fMRI block design with BOLD imaging. Social Cognitive and Affective Neuroscience, 11(3), 496. https://doi.org/10.1093/scan/nsv133

The Blue Zones: Buettner, D. (2010). The Blue Zones: Lessons for Living Longer from the People Who've Lived the Longest. National Geographic Society.

Stronger purpose in life is associated with decreased all-cause mortality: Alimujiang, A., Wiensch, A., Boss, J., Fleischer, N. L., Mondul, A. M., McLean, K., Mukherjee, B., & Pearce, C. L. (2019). Association Between Life Purpose and Mortality Among US Adults Older Than 50 Years. JAMA network open, 2(5), e194270. https://doi.org/10.1001/jamanetworkopen.2019.4270

The Ohsaki Study: Sone, T., Nakaya, N., Ohmori, K., Shimazu, T., Higashiguchi, M., Kakizaki, M., Kikuchi, N., Kuriyama, S., & Tsuji, I. (2008). Sense of life worth living (ikigai) and mortality in Japan: Ohsaki Study. Psychosomatic medicine, 70(6), 709–715. https://doi.org/10.1097/PSY.0b013e31817e7e64

Meaning rewires the brain: healthNair, A. K., Adluru, N., Finley, A. J., Gresham, L. K., Skinner, S. E., Alexander, A. L., Davidson, R. J., Ryff, C. D., & Schaefer, S. M. (2024). Purpose in life as a resilience factor for brain health: diffusion MRI findings from the Midlife in the U.S. study. Frontiers in psychiatry, 15, 1355998. https://doi.org/10.3389/fpsyt.2024.1355998

People with a strong sense of purpose have heightened activity in the prefrontal cortex: D'Argembeau A. (2013). On the role of the ventromedial prefrontal cortex in self-processing: the valuation hypothesis. Frontiers in human neuroscience, 7, 372. https://doi.org/10.3389/fnhum.2013.00372

Older adults with a high sense of purpose in life exhibit better cognitive function despite the burden of Alzheimer's disease: Boyle, P. A., Buchman, A. S., Wilson, R. S., Yu, L., Schneider, J. A., & Bennett, D. A. (2012). Effect of purpose in life on the relation between Alzheimer disease pathologic changes on cognitive function in advanced age. Archives of general psychiatry, 69(5), 499–505. https://doi.org/10.1001/archgenpsychiatry.2011.1487

Default mode network: Garrison, K. A., Zeffiro, T. A., Scheinost, D., Constable, R. T., & Brewer, J. A. (2015). Meditation leads to reduced default mode network activity beyond an active task. Cognitive, Affective & Behavioral Neuroscience, 15(3), 712. https://doi.org/10.3758/s13415-015-0358-3

Individuals who reported a high sense of purpose had significantly lower levels of C-reactive protein (CRP): Guimond, A. J., Shiba, K., Kim, E. S., & Kubzansky, L. D. (2022). Sense of purpose in life and inflammation in healthy older adults: A longitudinal study. Psychoneuroendocrinology, 141, 105746. https://doi.org/10.1016/j.psyneuen.2022.105746

Purpose extends our lifespan: Hill, P. L., & Turiano, N. A. (2014). Purpose in life as a predictor of mortality across adulthood. Psychological science, 25(7), 1482–1486. https://doi.org/10.1177/0956797614531799

Oxytocin: Mehdi, S. F., Pusapati, S., Khenhrani, R. R., Farooqi, M. S., Sarwar, S., Alnasarat, A., Mathur, N., Metz, C. N., LeRoith, D., Tracey, K. J., Yang, H., Brownstein, M. J., & Roth, J. (2022). Oxytocin and Related Peptide Hormones: Candidate Anti-Inflammatory Therapy in Early Stages of Sepsis. Frontiers in Immunology, 13, 864007. https://doi.org/10.3389/fimmu.2022.864007

Purpose, prosocial behaviors: Walker, C. S., Li, L., Baracchini, G., Tremblay-Mercier, J., Spreng, R. N., PREVENT-AD Research Group, & Geddes, M. R. (2023). The influence of generativity on purpose in life is mediated by social support and moderated by prefrontal functional connectivity in at-risk older adults. bioRxiv : the preprint server for biology, 2023.02.26.530089. https://doi.org/10.1101/2023.02.26.530089

Purpose, prosocial behaviors: Lee E. E. (2023). Relationships of Purpose in Life with Mental Health Among Older Adults: Links to Health and Social Behaviors. The American journal of geriatric psychiatry : official journal of the American Association for Geriatric Psychiatry, 31(2), 94–96. https://doi.org/10.1016/j.jagp.2022.10.001

Self-esteem is crucial for forming healthy relationships: Harris, M. A., & Orth, U. (2020). The link between self-esteem and social relationships: A meta-analysis of longitudinal studies. Journal of personality and social psychology, 119(6), 1459–1477. https://doi.org/10.1037/pspp0000265

Chapter 6

Interdependence: Covey, S. R. (1989). The 7 habits of highly effective people: Powerful lessons in personal change. Free Press.

The Blue Zones: Buettner, D. (2010). The Blue Zones: Lessons for Living Longer from the People

Who've Lived the Longest. National Geographic Society.

The Hadza: Pontzer, H., Wood, B. M., & Raichlen, D. A. (2018). Hunter-gatherers as models in public health. Obesity reviews : an official journal of the International Association for the Study of Obesity, 19 Suppl 1, 24–35. https://doi.org/10.1111/obr.12785

Okinawan moai: Buettner, D., & Skemp, S. (2016). Blue Zones: Lessons From the World's Longest Lived. American journal of lifestyle medicine, 10(5), 318–321. https://doi.org/10.1177/1559827616637066

Social connections are a cornerstone of health and longevity: Holt-Lunstad, J., Smith, T. B., & Layton, J. B. (2010). Social relationships and mortality risk: a meta-analytic review. PLoS medicine, 7(7), e1000316. https://doi.org/10.1371/journal.pmed.1000316

Community and longevity: Gronewold, J., Kropp, R., Lehmann, N., Schmidt, B., Weyers, S., Siegrist, J., Dragano, N., Jöckel, K. H., Erbel, R., Hermann, D. M., & Heinz Nixdorf Recall Study Investigative Group (2020). Association of social relationships with incident cardiovascular events and all-cause mortality. Heart (British Cardiac Society), 106(17), 1317–1323. https://doi.org/10.1136/heartjnl-2019-316250

The human brain is not designed for isolation: Holt-Lunstad, J., Smith, T. B., Baker, M., Harris, T., & Stephenson, D. (2015). Loneliness and social isolation as risk factors for mortality: a meta-analytic review. Perspectives on psychological science : a journal of the Association for Psychological Science, 10(2), 227–237. https://doi.org/10.1177/1745691614568352

Loneliness and pain: Loeffler, A., & Steptoe, A. (2021). Bidirectional longitudinal associations between loneliness and pain, and the role of inflammation. Pain, 162(3), 930–937. https://doi.org/10.1097/j.pain.0000000000002082

Chronic social isolation is as lethal as smoking: Holt-Lunstad, J., Smith, T. B., Baker, M., Harris, T., & Stephenson, D. (2015). Loneliness and Social Isolation as Risk Factors for Mortality. Perspectives on Psychological Science. https://doi.org/10.1177/1745691614568352

Loneliness: D'Agostino, A. E., Kattan, D., & Canli, T. (2019). An fMRI study of loneliness in younger and older adults. Social neuroscience, 14(2), 136–148. https://doi.org/10.1080/17470919.2018.1445027

Intimate groups provide significant support against modern stressors: Li, F., Luo, S., Mu, W., Li, Y., Ye, L., Zheng, X., Xu, B., Ding, Y., Ling, P., Zhou, M., & Chen, X. (2021). Effects of sources of social support and resilience on the mental health of different age groups during the COVID-19 pandemic. BMC psychiatry, 21(1), 16. https://doi.org/10.1186/s12888-020-03012-1

Increased screen time correlates with higher rates of depression: Vidal, C., Lhaksampa, T., Miller, L., & Platt, R. (2020). Social media use and depression in adolescents: a scoping review. International review of psychiatry (Abingdon, England), 32(3), 235–253. https://doi.org/10.1080/09540261.2020.1720623

Oxytocin: Carter C. S. (2021). Oxytocin and love: Myths, metaphors and mysteries. Comprehensive psychoneuroendocrinology, 9, 100107. https://doi.org/10.1016/j.cpnec.2021.100107

Mirror neurons: Kilner, J., & Lemon, R. (2013). What We Know Currently about Mirror Neurons. Current Biology, 23(23), R1057. https://doi.org/10.1016/j.cub.2013.10.051

A key player in this social circuitry is the default mode network (DMN): Li, W., Mai, X., & Liu, C. (2014). The default mode network and social understanding of others: what do brain connectivity studies tell us. Frontiers in human neuroscience, 8, 74. https://doi.org/10.3389/fnhum.2014.00074

Social engagement, vagal tone: Porges S. W. (2009). The polyvagal theory: new insights into adaptive reactions of the autonomic nervous system. Cleveland Clinic journal of medicine, 76 Suppl 2(Suppl 2), S86–S90. https://doi.org/10.3949/ccjm.76.s2.17

Harvard's 75-year first-generation Study of Adult Development: Atherton, O. E., Graham, E. K., Dorame, A. N., Horgan, D., Luo, J., Nevarez, M. D., Ferrie, J. P., Spiro, A., Schulz, M. S., Waldinger, R. J., Mroczek, D. K., & Lee, L. O. (2023). Is there intergenerational continuity in early life experiences? Findings from the Harvard Study of Adult Development. Journal of family psychology : JFP : journal of the Division of Family Psychology of the American Psychological Association (Division 43), 37(8), 1123–1136. https://doi.org/10.1037/fam0001144

Spending money on others lifts our spirits more than spending on ourselves: Dunn, E. W., Aknin, L. B., & Norton, M. I. (2008). Spending money on others promotes happiness. Science (New York, N.Y.), 319(5870), 1687–1688. https://doi.org/10.1126/science.1150952

Social engagement is crucial: Martino J, Pegg J, Frates EP. The Connection Prescription: Using the Power of Social Interactions and the Deep Desire for Connectedness to Empower Health and Wellness. Am J Lifestyle Med. 2015 Oct 7;11(6):466-475. doi: 10.1177/1559827615608788. PMID: 30202372; PMCID: PMC6125010.

Frequent social interaction strengthens neural connections: Kumar, M., Muhammad, T., & Dwivedi, L. K. (2022). Assessing the role of depressive symptoms in the association between social engagement and cognitive functioning among older adults: analysis of cross-sectional data from the Longitudinal Aging Study in India (LASI). BMJ open, 12(10), e063336. https://doi.org/10.1136/bmjopen-2022-063336

Individuals with higher levels of purpose exhibited lower levels of neurodegenerative pathology: Abellaneda-Pérez, K., Cattaneo, G., Cabello-Toscano, M. et al. Purpose in life promotes resilience to age-related brain burden in middle-aged adults. Alz Res Therapy 15, 49 (2023). https://doi.org/10.1186/s13195-023-01198-6

Purpose and cognitive health: Pfund, G. N., Spears, I., Norton, S. A., Bogdan, R., Oltmanns, T. F., & Hill, P. L. (2022). Sense of purpose as a potential buffer between mental health and subjective cognitive decline. International psychogeriatrics, 34(12), 1045–1055. https://doi.org/10.1017/S1041610222000680

Acts of service, psychological benefits: Kail, B. L., & Carr, D. C. (2020). More Than Selection Effects: Volunteering Is Associated With Benefits in Cognitive Functioning. The journals of gerontology. Series B, Psychological sciences and social sciences, 75(8), 1741–1746. https://doi.org/10.1093/geronb/gbaa101

Regularly volunteering and partaking in altruistic activities have been linked to increased lifespan: Konrath, S., Fuhrel-Forbis, A., Lou, A., & Brown, S. (2012). Motives for volunteering are associated with mortality risk in older adults. Health psychology : official journal of the Division of Health Psychology, American Psychological Association, 31(1), 87–96. https://doi.org/10.1037/a0025226

Epigenetics of bonding: Moon, A. L., Clifton, N. E., Wellard, N., Thomas, K. L., Hall, J., & Brydges, N. M. (2022). Social interaction following prepubertal stress alters prefrontal gene expression associated with cell signalling and oligodendrocytes. Translational psychiatry, 12(1), 516. https://doi.org/10.1038/s41398-022-02280-7

Epigenetics of bonding: Laubach, Z. M., Greenberg, J. R., Turner, J. W., Montgomery, T. M., Pioon, M. O., Sawdy, M. A., Smale, L., Cavalcante, R. G., Padmanabhan, K. R., Lalancette, C., vonHoldt, B., Faulk, C. D., Dolinoy, D. C., Holekamp, K. E., & Perng, W. (2021). Early-life social experience affects offspring DNA methylation and later life stress phenotype. Nature communications, 12(1), 4398. https://doi.org/10.1038/s41467-021-24583-x

Benefits of collective healing: Schleyer, W., Zona, K., Quigley, D., & Spottswood, M. (2022). Group therapy in primary care settings for the treatment of posttraumatic stress disorder: A systematic literature review. General hospital psychiatry, 77, 1–10. https://doi.org/10.1016/j.genhosppsych.2022.03.010

Benefits of collective healing: Asano, K., Tsuchiya, M., Okamoto, Y., Ohtani, T., Sensui, T., Masuyama, A., Isato, A., Shoji, M., Shiraishi, T., Shimizu, E., Irons, C., & Gilbert, P. (2022). Benefits of group compassion-focused therapy for treatment-resistant depression: A pilot randomized controlled trial. Frontiers in psychology, 13, 903842. https://doi.org/10.3389/fpsyg.2022.903842

Limbic resonance: Carr, L., Iacoboni, M., Dubeau, M. C., Mazziotta, J. C., & Lenzi, G. L. (2003). Neural mechanisms of empathy in humans: a relay from neural systems for imitation to limbic areas. Proceedings of the National Academy of Sciences of the United States of America, 100(9), 5497–5502. https://doi.org/10.1073/pnas.0935845100

Emotional contagion: Christakis, N. A., & Fowler, J. H. (2013). Social contagion theory: examining dynamic social networks and human behavior. Statistics in medicine, 32(4), 556–577. https://doi.org/10.1002/sim.5408

Emotional contagion: Prochazkova, E., & Kret, M. E. (2017). Connecting minds and sharing emotions through mimicry: A neurocognitive model of emotional contagion. Neuroscience and biobehavioral reviews, 80, 99–114. https://doi.org/10.1016/j.neubiorev.2017.05.013

Shared moods and health: Yamashita, Y., & Yamamoto, T. (2021). Perceiving Positive Facial Expression Can Relieve Depressive Moods: The Effect of Emotional Contagion on Mood in People With Subthreshold Depression. Frontiers in psychology, 12, 535980. https://doi.org/10.3389/fpsyg.2021.535980

Shared moods and health: Kuang, B., Peng, S., Wu, Y., Chen, Y., & Hu, P. (2023). The Neural Mechanisms of Group Membership Effect on Emotional Mimicry: A Multimodal Study Combining Electromyography and Electroencephalography. Brain sciences, 14(1), 25. https://doi.org/10.3390/brainsci14010025

Chapter 7

Epeme men: Marlowe, F. W. (2010). The Hadza: Hunter-Gatherers of Tanzania. Univ. of California Press.

Bicentennial Man: Columbus, C. (Director). (1999). Bicentennial man [Film]. Touchstone Pictures.

The infinite game: Sinek, S. (2019). The infinite game. Portfolio/Penguin.

Individuals who accept and embrace their finite nature often report making healthier life decisions: Yufe, S. J., Fergus, K. D., & Male, D. A. (2019). Lifestyle change experiences among breast cancer survivors participating in a pilot intervention: A narrative thematic analysis. European journal of oncology nursing : the official journal of European Oncology Nursing Society, 41, 97–103. https://doi.org/10.1016/j.ejon.2019.06.001

Existential psychology: Wong P. T. P. (2020). Existential positive psychology and integrative meaning therapy. International review of psychiatry (Abingdon, England), 32(7-8), 565–578. https://doi.org/10.1080/09540261.2020.1814703

Existential psychology: Mayer C. H. (2022). Positive and Existential Psychology in Times of Change: Towards Complex, Holistic, Systemic, and Integrative Perspectives. International journal of environmental research and public health, 19(14), 8433. https://doi.org/10.3390/ijerph19148433

Acknowledging mortality: Churchill L. R. (2023). Accepting and Embracing Our Mortality. Perspectives in biology and medicine, 66(3), 451–460. https://doi.org/10.1353/pbm.2023.a902037

Acknowledging mortality: Baars J. (2017). Aging: Learning to Live a Finite Life. The Gerontologist, 57(5), 969–976. https://doi.org/10.1093/geront/gnw089

Cosmic awe: Monroy, M., Uğurlu, Ö., Zerwas, F., Corona, R., Keltner, D., Eagle, J., & Amster, M. (2023). The influences of daily experiences of awe on stress, somatic health, and well-being: a longitudinal study during COVID-19. Scientific reports, 13(1), 9336. https://doi.org/10.1038/s41598-023-35200-w

Existential vacuum: Frankl, V. E. (2006). Man's search for meaning (I. Lasch, Trans.). Beacon Press. (Original work published 1946)

Oneness: Thuan T. X. (2001). Cosmic design from a Buddhist perspective. Annals of the New York Academy of Sciences, 950, 206–214. https://doi.org/10.1111/j.1749-6632.2001.tb02139.x

Oneness: Easwaran, E. (Trans.). (2007). The Upanishads (2nd ed.). Nilgiri Press.

Compassion meditation: Di Fabio, A., & Saklofske, D. H. (2021). The relationship of compassion and self-compassion with personality and emotional intelligence. Personality and individual differences, 169, 110109. https://doi.org/10.1016/j.paid.2020.110109

Compassion meditation: Graser, J., & Stangier, U. (2018). Compassion and Loving-Kindness Meditation: An Overview and Prospects for the Application in Clinical Samples. Harvard review of psychiatry, 26(4), 201–215. https://doi.org/10.1097/HRP.0000000000000192

Mindfulness and gene expression: Black, D. S., Christodoulou, G., & Cole, S. (2019). Mindfulness meditation and gene expression: a hypothesis-generating framework. Current opinion in psychology, 28, 302–306. https://doi.org/10.1016/j.copsyc.2019.06.004

Quantum entanglement: Einstein A, Podolsky B, Rosen N. Can quantum-mechanical description of physical reality be considered complete? Phys Rev. 1935;47:777–780. doi: 10.1103/PhysRev.47.777.

Creative work, cognitive reserve: Mashinchi, G. M., McFarland, C. P., Hall, S., Strongin, D. L., Williams, G. A., & Cotter, K. A. (2024). Handicraft art leisure activities and cognitive reserve. The

Clinical neuropsychologist, 38(3), 683–714. https://doi.org/10.1080/13854046.2023.2253993

The force of renewal and vitality: Song, S., Stern, Y., & Gu, Y. (2022). Modifiable lifestyle factors and cognitive reserve: A systematic review of current evidence. Ageing research reviews, 74, 101551. https://doi.org/10.1016/j.arr.2021.101551

The less we are the more life is: Sadhguru. (2016). Inner engineering: A yogi's guide to joy. Spiegel & Grau.

Aging and cellular decline: Cadenas, E., & Davies, K. J. (2000). Mitochondrial free radical generation, oxidative stress, and aging. Free radical biology & medicine, 29(3-4), 222–230. https://doi.org/10.1016/s0891-5849(00)00317-8

Renewal and vitality, hormesis: Santoro, A., Martucci, M., Conte, M., Capri, M., Franceschi, C., & Salvioli, S. (2020). Inflammaging, hormesis and the rationale for anti-aging strategies. Ageing research reviews, 64, 101142. https://doi.org/10.1016/j.arr.2020.101142

Chapter 8

A plant-based, whole-food diet: Fernández-Fígares Jiménez M. D. C. (2025). A Whole Plant-Foods Diet in the Prevention and Treatment of Overweight and Obesity: From Empirical Evidence to Potential Mechanisms. Journal of the American Nutrition Association, 44(2), 137–155. https://doi.org/10.1080/27697061.2024.2406887

Neuroplasticity: Johnson, B. P., & Cohen, L. G. (2023). Applied strategies of neuroplasticity. Handbook of clinical neurology, 196, 599–609. https://doi.org/10.1016/B978-0-323-98817-9.00011-9

Metabolism myth: Pontzer, H., Yamada, Y., Sagayama, H., Ainslie, P. N., Andersen, L. F., Anderson, L. J., Arab, L., Baddou, I., Bedu-Addo, K., Blaak, E. E., Blanc, S., Bonomi, A. G., Bouten, C. V. C., Bovet, P., Buchowski, M. S., Butte, N. F., Camps, S. G., Close, G. L., Cooper, J. A., Cooper, R., ... IAEA DLW Database Consortium (2021). Daily energy expenditure through the human life course. Science (New York, N.Y.), 373(6556), 808–812. https://doi.org/10.1126/science.abe5017

Mycobacterium vaccae can even act as a natural antidepressant: Foxx, C. L., Heinze, J. D., González, A., Vargas, F., Baratta, M. V., Elsayed, A. I., Stewart, J. R., Loupy, K. M., Arnold, M. R., Flux, M. C., Sago, S. A., Siebler, P. H., Milton, L. N., Lieb, M. W., Hassell, J. E., Smith, D. G., K Lee, K. A., Appiah, S. A., Schaefer, E. J., . . . Lowry, C. A. (2021). Effects of Immunization With the Soil-Derived Bacterium Mycobacterium vaccae on Stress Coping Behaviors and Cognitive Performance in a "Two Hit" Stressor Model. Frontiers in Physiology, 11, 524833. https://doi.org/10.3389/fphys.2020.524833

Chapter 9

Physiologically, a lower respiratory rate is directly correlated with increased parasympathetic tone: Zaccaro, A., Piarulli, A., Laurino, M., Garbella, E., Menicucci, D., Neri, B., & Gemignani, A. (2018). How Breath-Control Can Change Your Life: A Systematic Review on Psycho-Physiological Correlates of Slow Breathing. Frontiers in human neuroscience, 12, 353. https://doi.org/10.3389/fnhum.2018.00353

Longest living creatures, respiratory rates: Berta, A., Sumich, J. L., & Kovacs, K. M. (2015). Marine mammals: Evolutionary biology (3rd ed.). Academic Press.

The Greenland shark: Nielsen, J., Hedeholm, R. B., Heinemeier, J., Bushnell, P. G., Christiansen, J. S., Olsen, J., Ramsey, C. B., Brill, R. W., Simon, M., Steffensen, K. F., & Steffensen, J. F. (2016). Eye lens radiocarbon reveals centuries of longevity in the Greenland shark (Somniosus microcephalus). Science (New York, N.Y.), 353(6300), 702–704. https://doi.org/10.1126/science.aaf1703

DISCLAIMER

The information in *Primal Health Design: 7 Key Paradigms to Reverse Biological Age* is intended for general educational and lifestyle guidance purposes only. It reflects the author's personal opinions, experiences, and research and is not a substitute for professional medical advice, diagnosis, or treatment.

This book is not designed to diagnose, treat, cure, or prevent any disease. If you have, or suspect that you have, a medical condition, including but not limited to cardiovascular disease, diabetes, cancer, or respiratory issues, you should consult a licensed healthcare provider before implementing any of the practices, dietary changes, or exercise routines mentioned in this book.

All readers are encouraged to work in partnership with their qualified healthcare team. The author and publisher expressly disclaim any responsibility for adverse effects that may result from using or applying the information contained in this book.

We hope that the insights and practices shared here serve as a supportive addition to your overall health strategy, complementing the care and recommendations provided by your primary care physician and medical team.

ABOUT THE AUTHOR

Dr. Kavin Mistry is a board-certified neuroradiologist, medical educator, health author, and speaker. He is trained in Age Management Medicine, which combines the latest scientific advancements with ancestral health wisdom to help individuals reverse biological aging and thrive in today's world. Dr. Mistry serves as core faculty for radiology residents and medical students in the greater Philadelphia area and is highly respected for his thoughtful, interdisciplinary approach to health and education.

Dr. Mistry has been recognized among South Jersey Magazine's Top Docs and has authored peer-reviewed work in journals such as the *American Journal of Roentgenology*. His research in neuroimaging and neuroscience has been presented at leading national conferences including the Radiological Society of North America (RSNA) and Society for Imaging Informatics in Medicine (SIIM).

His approach to health is deeply personal and shaped by a rich global upbringing. During his childhood years in Tanzania, Africa, he spent time with the Hadzabe tribe, one of the world's last remaining hunter-gatherer communities. There, he developed an early appreciation for the rhythms of nature and the primal intelligence of the human body. Raised in a traditional Indian household, he was equally immersed in Eastern philosophies, Ayurvedic practices, and a holistic worldview. He also descends from a lineage of master woodworkers, a background that instilled in him a respect for craftsmanship, harmony, and the healing power of design.

A dynamic speaker and thought leader, Dr. Mistry has delivered talks on stroke imaging, high-performance living, and holistic lifestyle transformation. His work bridges high-tech medical innovation with time-honored health principles, guiding readers to awaken vitality, extend healthspan, and reconnect with their biological and spiritual roots.

Primal Health Design is both a synthesis of his journey and a blueprint for yours—an invitation to live younger, stronger, and more aligned with your true nature.

Connect with Dr. Mistry and explore more resources at:

KavinMistryMD.com

PrimalHealthDesign.com

PrimalResetProgram.com

www.ingramcontent.com/pod-product-compliance
Lightning Source LLC
Chambersburg PA
CBHW080416030426
42335CB00020B/2475